Perspectives in Nursing Management and Care for Older Adults

Series Editors

Julie Santy-Tomlinson
School of Health Sciences
University of Manchester
Manchester, UK

Paolo Falaschi
Sant'Andrea Hospital
Sapienza University of Rome
Rome, Italy

Karen Hertz
University Hospitals of North Midlands
Royal Stoke University Hospital
Stoke-on-Trent, Staffordshire, UK

The aim of this book series is to provide a comprehensive guide to nursing management and care for older adults, addressing specific problems in nursing and allied health professions. It provides a unique resource for nurses, enabling them to provide high-quality care for older adults in all care settings. The respective volumes are designed to provide practitioners with highly accessible information on evidence-based management and care for older adults, with a focus on practical guidance and advice.

Though demographic trends in developed countries are sometimes assumed to be limited to said countries, it is clear that similar issues are now affecting rapidly developing countries in Asia and South America. As such, the series will not only benefit nurses working in Europe, North America, Australasia and many developed countries, but also elsewhere. Offering seminal texts for nurses working with older adults in both inpatient and outpatient settings, it will especially support them during the first five years after nurse registration, as they move towards specialist and advanced practice. The series will also be of value to student nurses, employing a highly accessible style suitable for a broader readership.

More information about this series at http://www.springer.com/series/15860

Wilfred McSherry • Linda Rykkje
Susan Thornton

Editors

Understanding Ageing for Nurses and Therapists

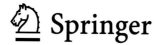 Springer

Editors
Wilfred McSherry
Department of Nursing
School of Health and Social Care
Staffordshire University
Stoke-On-Trent
UK

University Hospitals of North
Midlands NHS Trust
Stoke-on-Trent/Stafford
England
UK

Professor VID Specialized University
College Bergen/Oslo
Oslo
Norway

Linda Rykkje
Faculty of Health Studies
VID Specialized University
Bergen
Norway

Susan Thornton
Department of Nursing
School of Health and Social Care
Centre of Excellence in Healthcare Education
Staffordshire University
Shrewsbury
UK

ISSN 2522-8838   ISSN 2522-8846   (electronic)
Perspectives in Nursing Management and Care for Older Adults
ISBN 978-3-030-40074-3   ISBN 978-3-030-40075-0   (eBook)
https://doi.org/10.1007/978-3-030-40075-0

This Springer imprint is published by the registered company Springer Nature Switzerland AG
The registered company address is: Gewerbestrasse 11, 6330 Cham, Switzerland

Foreword

You can live to be a hundred if you give up all things that make you want to live to be a hundred.
—Woody Allen

It has always been of interest to me that any discussions of 'ageing' are actually discussions of 'older age' as most commentators, writers and indeed researchers seem to (implicitly at least) imply that ageing begins at 50! The reality that ageing starts from the moment we are born (or perhaps even before, depending on your belief system!) seems to bypass thinking in this field. As a result, society is organically ageist as there seems to be no accepted discourse for ageing during early years and early adulthood. The discourses for this period of life are instead dominated by psychological and sociological developmental theories, as if this period of life was preparation for a period of ageing that is yet to be experienced. Of course, as we all know, it is these formative years that shape all those that follow and so how we psychologically, sociologically, spiritually and physically age as younger persons has a profound impact on our overall ageing trajectory. So, any book that sets out to address ageing is inevitably caught up in this dilemma of 'where to begin' because in reality a book about ageing is a book about the life course from birth to death!

The authors of *Understanding Ageing for Nurses and Therapists* of course are faced with an additional dilemma—Covid-19. At the time the book goes to print we are still all gripped with the challenges of finding our way out of this global pandemic. Whilst some countries have fared better than others in terms of the numbers of people who have died from the virus, no country has been able to avoid it. Common to all our collective experience has been the impact that the coronavirus has on older people and especially those with multiple morbidities and residing in care homes. At times this has been distressing to observe and difficult to accept the consequences that so many older people, their families and friends have had to endure. But of course, what the coronavirus has managed to do is shine a very bright light on differences across the generations and the impact of different experiences of ageing across the life course. Whilst young adults can celebrate the fact that the virus is less likely to make them sick than older adults, they also carry a huge burden of responsibility to not act as 'super-spreaders' as asymptomatic carriers of the virus. As someone who has worked in the field of ageing for most of my professional life, the differences I have observed among age groups during the pandemic have been interesting and intriguing—for example, attitudes towards social distancing and behaviours associated with wearing face coverings. As I engaged in my daily exercise regime during 'lockdown periods' it was interesting to me how older and younger adults considered the importance or otherwise of things like social distancing and the fairly cavalier attitude towards it among younger compared with older adults. 'The invincibility of youth' is a well-worn phrase, and in this example it would be easy to be dismissive of younger people as 'not caring enough', but perhaps we need to re-frame such judgements. Perhaps it is because of the invincibility of youth that healthy ageing is possible at all, as the author John Green asserts in his book, *Looking for Alaska*:

> *When adults say, "Teenagers think they are invincible" with that sly, stupid smile on their faces, they don't know how right they are. We need never be hopeless, because we can never be irreparably broken. We think that we are invincible because we are. We cannot be born, and we cannot die. Like all energy, we can only change shapes and sizes and manifestations. They forget that when they get old. They get scared of losing and failing. But that part of us greater than the sum of our parts cannot begin and cannot end, and so it cannot fail. (p 220)*

Green articulates with some degree of irony the energy required to age with some degree of success (whatever that really means!). The fact that so many people live to a grand old age is the success of our time, which not even coronavirus can stop! The intricate configuration of physiological, sociological, psychological, spiritual and relational factors, which together with sheer bloody-mindedness and immense energy for living, means we successfully traverse the life course. The authors of *Understanding Ageing for Nurses and Therapists* 'get' this and have constructed a text that is not dominated by the vagaries of the ageing mind and body, but instead articulates this intricate configuration and the need to continuously update our beliefs, attitudes and evidence.

I am also conscious though that we can paint a picture of ageing that is pollyannaish, whilst the lived experience for many persons is quite the opposite. For some people, their life course is blighted by various challenges that means there is an imbalance between the energy needed to traverse the life course 'healthily' and the resources available to them to do so. As a gerontological nurse, I have always been very conscious of this in my practice and one of the reasons why I feel so passionately about the adoption of person-centred approaches. The older person in need of care is someone who has managed to successfully bring sustained energy to their life course, but who in the end has a need for the input of others to help them make it through to the end. We can either see this as a failure of our body systems to sustain the energy needed to manage the intricacies of life or we can see it as a natural progression from the 'invincible independence' of youth to the 'insuperable interdependence' of older age.

The chapters of this book take us through this journey and hold the space for us to layer our own understandings and interpretations of this lifelong journey. As Green asserts, it enables us to '… *change shapes and sizes and manifestations*'. At a time when the complexities and intricacies of ageing are more challenging than ever before, when the ongoing impact of global influences and challenges are better understood and when society is increasingly challenged to shift its norms, then considering how to age well through this is essential. This book makes an important contribution to this contemporary picture and will facilitate important debate and discussion among those who engage with the text.

Brendan McCormack
Divisions of Nursing, Occupational Therapy and Art Therapies
Centre for Person-Centred Practice Research, Queen Margaret University
Edinburgh, Scotland

Omega XI Chapter, Sigma Global
Edinburgh, Scotland

Reference

1. Green J (2005) Looking for Alaska. Harper Collins, London

Contents

Introduction: Understand Ageing and How We Care for Older People—Reflections, Legacy and Lessons Learned in the Wake of COVID-19

1

Wilfred McSherry, Linda Rykkje, and Susan Thornton

Contents

W. McSherry (✉)
Department of Nursing, School of Health and Social Care, Staffordshire University, Stoke-On-Trent, UK

University Hospitals of North Midlands NHS Trust, Stoke-on-Trent/Stafford, England, UK

Professor VID Specialized University College Bergen/Oslo, Oslo, Norway
e-mail: w.mcsherry@staffs.ac.uk

L. Rykkje
Faculty of Health Studies, VID Specialized University, Bergen, Norway
e-mail: linda.rykkje@vid.no

S. Thornton
Department of Nursing, School of Health and Social Care, Centre of Excellence in Healthcare Education, Staffordshire University, Shrewsbury, UK

© Springer Nature Switzerland AG 2021
W. McSherry et al. (eds.), *Understanding Ageing for Nurses and Therapists*,
Perspectives in Nursing Management and Care for Older Adults,
https://doi.org/10.1007/978-3-030-40075-0_1

Understanding the normal ageing processes and mechanisms is of vital importance for all nursing and allied health and social care professions. This will support them when providing care for older people, their families and friends across diverse health and social care sectors. The primary goal of this text is to explore some of the neglected contemporary issues associated with ageing such as spirituality, sexuality, death and dying. The aim is to break down barriers and dispel some of the myths and misconceptions that are often perpetuated across generations, within professions and throughout care settings.

Given that the epidemiological evidence indicates many people are now living longer and healthier lives it is imperative that those caring for older people have a sound knowledge base of what normal ageing involves and how this may affect people physically, psychologically, socially and spiritually. Conversely, this knowledge will enable them to identify abnormal and pathological deviations from the norm allowing for a timely intervention. This type of knowledge will enable nurses and allied health and social care professionals to be more confident and competent in their care, being prepared to challenge and escalate concerns should these arise during their practice. It will also enable them to celebrate and share good practice across the different sectors.

1.1   Demographics and Context

One of the significant achievements of our health and social care systems across the world is the positive impact this has had upon life expectancy. For example, in the United Kingdom (UK) the Office for National Statistics [1] tells us that "In 2018, there were 13,170 centenarians (people aged 100 years and over) in the UK…"

From these figures we can assume that there are more people alive in the world today over the age of a hundred than at any point in human history. Roser et al. [2] indicate since the 1900s the global average life expectancy has more than doubled and is now above 70 years. Yet they are keen to stress despite these improvements inequalities around life expectancy persist across and within many countries. The above figures are also reflected by The United Nations [3, p. 9] which states

> While life expectancy at birth has improved, the improvement in life expectancy at older ages has been even more rapid. … Globally, a person who is turning 65 years old could expect to live an additional 17 years in 2015–2020, and this number could rise to 19 years in 2045–2050

Whilst these improvements in life expectancy are very welcome, it has presented a major challenge to societies around how we provide high quality and dignified care for our ageing populations. It must be stressed that these improvements in life-expectancy relate primarily to high- and middle-income countries and do not reflect the global picture where life expectancy can be much lower in some of the developing nations. Interestingly, some of the issues and challenges we face when caring for older people have been highlighted by the recent global pandemic.

1.2 A Global Pandemic

By way of introduction to this section we would like to express our utmost respect and gratitude to all health and social care colleagues across the world for their selfless sacrifice in the face of one of this century's greatest challenges. As we moved towards the completion and publication of this manuscript, the world is caught up in the grip of a global pandemic, COVID-19 coronavirus.

We have reflected on this very tragic situation and written part of this introduction around some of the key issues that illustrate and reinforce societies attitudes and understanding of ageing and crucially how we care for our older people. Because many of the issues we have experienced in this unprecedented and challenging time have had serious and catastrophic consequences for all of us but especially so for many of our older people.

The outbreak of this virus is purported to have originated in Wuhan the capital of Hubei province in the People's Republic of China. Due to several factors, globalisation, and international travel the virus spread rapidly across the globe affecting every continent, country, and peoples. The impact of this pandemic has been unprecedented, with millions of people dying, being hospitalised and in need of specialist critical care placing tremendous pressure on our health and social care services resulting in these being stretched to within breaking point. The rhetoric and imagery used by many countries resulted in the pandemic being described as a war with the mobilisation of resources, funding, and people to support the 'war effort'.

The pandemic has brought the best and the worst of humanities values, attitudes, and behaviours to the fore. Health and social care professionals have displayed heroism and resolve to preserve life and provide the best possible care including end of life in very challenging circumstance. They have done this with professionalism, altruism and compassion doing this behind personal protective equipment with dignity, sensitivity and in a spirit of unity and resolve. There is no escaping that the impact of the virus has been devastating with immediate and far reaching consequences for our health and social care systems, economies, and the future stability of many societies.

We have witnessed an existential disruption at a global level and the shattering, fracturing of everything that is meaningful and that adds value to the daily rituals' routines of everyday life. The term 'lockdown' has seen all of us in a state of self-isolation, with some of the most vulnerable in our communities, having no or limited contact with families, friends, and communities. Many things that we have taken for granted, often the ordinary and mundane are being re-evaluated; our work, relationships, and freedom. Consequently, many people are appraising their beliefs and values approaching life with new insight and a spiritual lens.

Despite some of the negativity, individuals, communities, and societies have united, come together and shown determination and solidarity. There have been many valiant acts of charity and selflessness to support those in need and specifically our older people. Health and social care professional have died while caring for those infected with COVID-19 and in need of life saving interventions. The public have rallied and shown great appreciation as expressed in the "Clap for carers" which is an international phenomenon, occurring in many European countries and further afield for example in the USA.

1.3   Older People Inspiring a Generation

During the Pandemic there have been many accounts of older people across the globe inspiring us with their acts of altruism. One of the most memorable moments in the UK was the late Sir Capt. Tom Moore at the age of 99 walking 100 laps of his garden before his 100th birthday to raise £1000 for the NHS. The public were moved with pride and admiration and by the 30th April the day of his birthday now Colonel Moore had raised a staggering £32,796,155 for NHS Charities Together (See https://www.justgiving.com/fundraising/tomswalkforthenhs).

In contrast we have heard of many older people dying in residential and nursing homes, where care staff have had limited or no access to personal protective equipment and testing. With many of these deaths of older people not even being recorded in the daily counts or having COVID-19 recorded on their death certificates. In the United Kingdom this was an outrage with commentators saying older people were being *'airbrushed'* out of the data [4]. It also raised some very fundamental questions about societies perceptions of older people highlighting that age discrimination still exists in many forms both explicitly and implicitly.

1.4   Norway Chooses a Different Approach

Norway has chosen a different approach to reduce the spread of the virus, and early on nursing homes were closed for visitors including close family. With a low total of deaths compared to other countries, the government has decided to gradually re-open parts of the society and allow socializing in smaller groups. However, (at the time of writing this introduction, Mid 2020) nursing homes are still closed for visitors. Then, one might ask, what is worst? Being isolated and not seeing family and friends, or being put at risk of catching COVID-19? These discussions will continue, as we see that it is often the personnel and not visitors that spread the virus to residents. In many regions where the risk of infection is low, perhaps visitors should be allowed? Is it avoiding the disease that is most important, or quality of life for residents? These questions are important, however, the overall situation for older people is not really discussed in the Norwegian media. Fear of spreading the disease is the main concern, thus this might also be a form of discrimination. The situation is changing with a press release from the Norwegian Government dated 8/4/2020 indicating that the country is to lift COVID-19 restrictions gradually and cautiously.

1.5   Age Is Not an Indicator of Ability

Age also seemed to be an arbitrary or even a discriminatory factor in the ethical decisions around who should be ventilated or not. With speculation that those over the age of 60 in some countries were not eligible. While this type of criteria needs to be confirmed post-pandemic it affirms that misconceptions still persist that age alone correlates with quality of life and that those above a certain age are considered to have 'had their lot' and thereby worthy recipients of death. These types of attitude place little value on 'life' setting up a precedence that the older we are the more deserving of death. This is a form of eugenics that implies younger people are more superior (deserving of life) than are our inferior older population.

The World Health Organisation [5] when discussing ageing and health states the following:

> If people can experience these extra years of life in good health and if they live in a supportive environment, their ability to do the things they value will be little different from that of a younger person. If these added years are dominated by declines in physical and mental capacity, the implications for older people and for society are more negative.

This quotation underlines and acknowledges that age is not a reason for older people to engage in those activities that add value, meaning and purpose in life. It is the role of our societies to enable and support our older people to live healthy and fulfilled lives and to prevent decline in their physical and mental capacity. United for All Ages (2020) is one wonderful example of different age groups and generations from across society coming together to find solutions to issues that impact on peoples live.

1.6   Positive Attitudes Towards Ageing

Chochinov [6] emphasising the A, B, C, D of dignity conserving care asserts that positive Attitudes lead to positive Behaviours. When we are caring for older people and indeed each other our behaviours must always be Compassionate and the vehicle for achieving all of this is Dialogue. Dignity conserving care is not delivered through words alone but requires action and this action must always be intrinsic, looking at our own attitudes and how these may influence our values and behaviours. Magee et al. [7, p. 9] capture this need for action so clearly when they write "It is easier to make pronouncement about dignity than to ensure dignified care happens." It is the responsibility and duty of all of us who care for older people to be proactive challenge any attitudes, values and behaviours that may have negative consequences for the way we care for older people.

Similarly, we must be aware of those organisational, institutional, team and even individual attitudes, values and behaviours that may lead to the violations of people's dignity. These attitudes, values and behaviours can be insidious and very corrosive if not challenged and removed. One solution to this is to ensure our attitudes towards ageing are not informed by the negative images and stereotypes that infiltrate social media and can dominate in some cultures and societies. For example, we seem to live in an age where youth and beauty is worshipped and should be preserved at all costs. While natural ageing and growing old are abnormal and should be prevented at all costs. Health and social care professionals are in a very powerful position to influence change and present a more 'holistic' and normal understanding of ageing and the biological, psychological, social and spiritual processes that this entails.

One of the editors (WMc) was once asked *'When will you stop teaching and speaking about dignity in the care of older people?'* The reply was 'When there are no longer any violations of older people's dignity?'

It is self-evident from the pandemic that in the face of great adversity and threat, some societies and individuals can neglect and fail in their duty to safeguard the dignity and lives of our older people. While at the same time health and social care professionals are prepared to compromise their own health and wellbeing to defend the needs of those who are vulnerable.

Fear, the lack of resources and a failure to ensure that older people and health and social care staff are adequately protected, by providing the correct personal protective equipment and testing have been the subject of much debate and criticism.

Fear, ignorance and misconception lead to stereotyping, discrimination, and inequality in the way that we care for older people. One of the aims of this book is to ensure that health and social care professionals are given up to date knowledge and evidence that will inform their own practice, enabling them to recognise when the quality and standards of care are being compromised.

1.7   The Need for a Holistic and Person-Centred Approach

At the time of writing in the UK over 126,155 people have died within 28 days of being diagnosed with COVID-19 (many within care homes and community settings) and behind every statistic is a personal story and life narrative. Sadly, the death and loss of any person irrespective of age has far reaching consequences for their immediate loved ones, friends, and colleagues and indeed the wider community in which they live. Given the sad circumstances associated with these deaths, people separated from loved ones, isolated and alone in hospitals and being cared for by health and social care professional wearing PPE. The long term psychological and emotional impact may see spouses, partners, children, experiencing adverse reactions to the loss, grief, and bereavement they have experienced. Similarly, health and social care professional providing care in these very challenging situations may experience post-traumatic stress disorder and loss of mental well-being due to the prolonged exposure in such stressful and highly charged situations.

Never before has there been the need to ensure that the care provided by all health and social care professional is compassionate, dignified and truly person-centred and holistic that is ensuring the spiritual and existential dimensions of a person's life are acknowledged and supported.

1.8   Legacy and Lessons Learned

The COVID-19 pandemic highlights a vital need for sustained and immediate investment in how we fund our health and social care services. A key priority must be an evaluation of how we support some of the most vulnerable within our society who were most affected our older people. The challenges faced and the issues raised will no doubt, be debated for many years to come. However, one legacy that will remain, arising from the pandemic globally, are the controversies around the status of older people and how in some countries the slow response taken to safeguard them which was wholly inadequate. A major lesson is the need to be more proactive than reactive. Given the changing nature of the situation almost on a daily/weekly basis which will be the case for many countries as the pandemic unfolds. This means that it will be difficult to predict the exact course and outcome of the pandemic. Because countries have adopted different strategies for recording and tracking the trajectory of the virus depending upon cultural and political /national contexts will mean generalisations cannot be made, but the legacy and lessons learned will inevitably be universal.

1.9　Overview of the Book

Understanding Ageing for Nurses and Therapists is a practical resource for all those responsible for caring for older people across health and social care. It provides a comprehensive and holistic approach helping nurses, therapists, and social care professionals to better understand the impact of ageing upon the person and wider society. A unique feature of this text is the focus upon positive ageing and the attempt to dispel and challenge some of the myths, prejudices and negative attitudes that still prevail towards ageing and older people.

The book is structured around thirteen chapters, excluding the introduction. Each of the chapters have been written by specialists in their field and presented in an engaging and interactive style, they draw upon case studies and scenarios to maximize engagement developing your competence, by informing your knowledge, attitudes, and skills. Chapter 2 explores physiology and ageing considering why we age and what the underlying processes are, before considering the effects of ageing on the systems of the body. While Chap. 3 offers an insight into the nature, benefits, and potential applications of a life history approach within health and social care highlighting how this is central to promoting the health and wellbeing of older people. A neglected aspect of health and social care is the concept of spirituality. This controversial area is discussed in Chap. 4 which introduces different views on how spiritual and existential issues may be relevant for older people. The psychology of ageing is addressed in Chap. 5. This chapter discusses normal age-related changes in cognition, personality, emotions, coping and control. The author explores how such changes may affect the everyday life of older people. Chapter 6 introduces the reader to issues associated with the sexual health of older people. This chapter affirms that sexual health discussions are an essential part of the holistic assessment of health and social needs and should lead to interventions that ensure older people are able to enjoy their rights and live healthy sexual lives.

Preventing the deconditioning of older people is introduced within Chap. 7. The awareness of important timely interventions can maintain physical function along with general health and well-being. Therefore this chapter will explore concepts such as frailty and comorbidity and how these may impact on the care of older people. The importance of recognising delirium and depression and how nurses and therapist may respond are also considered.

The importance of nutrition and ageing are explored within Chap. 8. The chapter offers an overview of the key factors that contribute to malnutrition in older people, delving into the evidence base offering a practical approach to the prevention and treatment of malnutrition in older people. Issues related to the continuity of care for older people between the hospital and the community environment are outlined in Chap. 9. Consideration is given to matters such as inter-professional working and how this takes place along with a discussion of the roles and responsibilities of social work professionals.

Chapter 10 deals with the fundamental aspect of palliative and end of life care. Because of the taboos and fears that exist in many societies around death and dying this can be a neglected aspect of care. This chapter offers valuable insights into providing good palliative and end of life care with an overarching aim of dispelling ageism while offering new perspectives.

Globally one of the significant challenges that older people face are issues associated with loneliness. Chapter 11 introduces two important concepts in older persons care namely self-neglect and loneliness. The chapter explores a range of factors contributing to these and ways in which nurses and therapists can work with older people to address and alleviate these issues. The need for safeguarding older people is recognised as an integral part of care delivery. Therefore, Chap. 12 explores human rights in the context of ethical and legal frameworks and how these may be applied to the care of older people.

Chapter 13 introduces the reader to the importance of governance quality and inspection or review. These concepts and processes play an important role in ensuring high quality services for older people across the full spectrum of sectors. Robust governance and quality assurance process ensure that any concerns can be escalated to the appropriate people and the relevant authorities notified so remedial action can be taken to safeguard those receiving and providing care.

The delivery of care to older people is constantly changing with new technologies and innovations being developed that can enhance care while promoting independence. Chapter 14 explores how contemporary care may comprise of technology affirming how this may influence the power balance between the older person and those assisting them.

From the above overview it is evident that the text introduces the reader to key dimensions of what it is to be a person, physically, psychologically, socially and spiritually and how these contribute to the ageing process and can enhance the quality of life of older people.

Irrespective of whether one cares for older people in an acute hospital setting or domiciliary, home care. The material and content transcend health and social care boundaries, providing valuable, contemporary evidence that can inform and shape practice. Above all this text will encourage reflection, dialogue, and engagement with some fundamental aspects of ageing, challenging, attitudes, values, and behaviour so that a more positive and balanced insight towards ageing is fostered.

This book will develop self-awareness and will inform your professional practice so these are enriched and informed ensuring you have a holistic understanding of ageing enabling you to care for older people with compassion, dignity and respect.

References

1. Office for National Statistics (2019) Estimates of the very old, including centenarians, UK: 2002 to 2018. https://www.ons.gov.uk/peoplepopulationandcommunity/birthsdeathsandmarriages/ageing/bulletins/estimatesoftheveryoldincludingcentenarians/2002to2018. Accessed 5 May 2020
2. Roser M, Ortiz-Ospina E, Ritchie H (2020) Life expectancy. https://ourworldindata.org/life-expectancy. Accessed 5 May 2020
3. United Nations (2020) World population ageing 2019. https://www.un.org/en/development/desa/population/publications/pdf/ageing/WorldPopulationAgeing2019-Report.pdf. Accessed 5 May 2020
4. ITV News Report (2020) Coronavirus death toll 'airbrushing out' older people dying in care system. https://www.itv.com/news/2020-04-13/coronavirus-death-toll-airbrushing-out-older-people-dying-in-care-system/. Accessed 5 May 2020
5. World Health Organisation (2018) Ageing and health. https://www.who.int/news-room/fact-sheets/detail/ageing-and-health. Accessed 5 May 2020
6. Chochinov HM (2007) Dignity and the essence of medicine: the A, B, C, and D of dignity conserving care. Dignity British Medical Journal 335:184–187
7. Magee H, Parsons S, Askham J (2008) 'Measuring dignity in care for older people' a research report for Help the Aged. Help the Aged, London, p 9
8. Norwegian Government (2020) Norway to lift COVID-19 restrictions gradually and cautiously. Press release I Date: 08/04/2020 I No: 62/20. https://www.regjeringen.no/en/aktuelt/norway-to-lift-covid-19-restrictions-gradually-and-cautiously/id2697060/. Accessed 14 May 2020

Physiology and Ageing

2

Roger Watson

Contents

2.1 Learning Objectives

This chapter will enable you to:

- understand the underlying processes that lead to ageing,
- know the effects of ageing on the major systems of the body,
- explain why multipathology and multipharmacology are more common with ageing.

2.2 Introduction to the Topic

Chronological ageing begins at birth, and up to adolescence the body grows and develops to maturity. Somewhere in the mid-20s the process of ageing begins and continues throughout our life to the point of death. At the time of writing, there is no

R. Watson (✉)
Faculty of Health Sciences, University of Hull, Hull, East Yorkshire, UK
e-mail: r.watson@hull.ac.uk

© Springer Nature Switzerland AG 2021
W. McSherry et al. (eds.), *Understanding Ageing for Nurses and Therapists*,
Perspectives in Nursing Management and Care for Older Adults,
https://doi.org/10.1007/978-3-030-40075-0_2

way of stopping or reversing the ageing process. Whether it can be slowed down is uncertain but, clearly, some people seem to age more quickly than the others and that some people survive the ageing process better than others. Genetics plays a great part in our response to ageing, but environmental factors also influence our response to ageing.

Therefore, there is no such thing as 'normal' ageing. However, it is given that we all age and that there is an increasing need to understand the ageing process because more people are living longer. In this chapter, I will cover what is known about the ageing process from the physiological perspective, what is common to everyone who ages and what the consequences are. Ageing is not a disease and ageing is not necessarily associated with disease. Nevertheless, ageing is associated with disease to a greater extent, and the boundary line between the ageing process and disease is very hard to define. Therefore, while some consideration of the disease processes that are more common in ageing is inevitable, I wish to focus more on the usual aspects of ageing and to explain why some diseases are more common in advanced.

2.2.1 What Is Ageing?

Before reading this section, reflect on the following:

- What is your understanding of the ageing process?
- What effect do you think ageing has on the various physiological systems of the body?

We all have a general understanding of what ageing is; we see it in the people around us and we experience it ourselves. We see the signs of ageing and these are most visible in our skin—especially noticeable in our faces—and our hair. We also note that posture changes as people age, and they, generally, become less 'fit' in the physiological sense. Ultimately becoming slower with age and suffering some degree of memory loss. But these are the outward signs of ageing. In concert with these outward changes, which, in themselves, are very superficial and largely inconsequential, ageing is experienced by every system of the body. It is these changes which are more important, especially in terms of the interface between ageing and disease and, ultimately, in determining our lifespan. I will cover each system of the body below. A general description of the ageing process could be that, with time, our bodies lack the capacity and the resilience they once had. The governing concept in physiology is homeostasis—maintaining a constant internal environment. Homeostasis requires the integration of several physiological systems and exists to benefit all the systems and organs in the body, but ensuring that fundamental properties such as body heat, hydration and the acid-base balance—amongst other things—do not move too far or for too long from the optimum levels at which they function best. With age, we become less able to maintain this constant internal environment. Within limits, this is not a problem to most people as they age; however, extremes of temperature, dehydration or any other physiological challenges are coped with less well by older people. We all have considerable reserve capacity in our bodies, but that reserve capacity declines with age [1]. It is especially noticeable in disease states, which can mount extreme physiological challenges to the body; generally speaking, younger people cope better with common diseases than older people.

2.2.2 Why Do We Age?

Why we age physiologically can be viewed in two ways:

- What is the reason for ageing (i.e. why do we not remain forever young?)?
- What are the underlying processes that lead to ageing?

2.2.2.1 What Is the Reason for Ageing?

Considering the reasons for ageing brings us into the realm of theories of ageing. There have been many theories of ageing and in some, such as the 'wear and tear theory', it is hard to distinguish cause and effect, and these do not really explain why the phenomenon of physiological ageing takes place. Other theories attempt to explain the need for ageing and why we do not remain young and, indeed, to live forever. Ageing is only really observed in humans and domestic animals. Few other animals age in the same sense as they rarely survive to experience it. Humans, on the other hand, have managed to extend their lifespans through nutritional, sanitary and medical advances and have inflicted old age on their domestic animals for similar reasons. Moreover, although it is generally accepted that there is a maximum possible lifespan of around 125 years (https://en.wikipedia.org/wiki/Maximum_life_span; accessed 20 November 2019), the 'normal' human lifespan is around 79 years (https://www.factinate.com/things/50-interesting-facts-human-body/; accessed 20 November 2019). Life expectancy (https://en.wikipedia.org/wiki/Life_expectancy; accessed 20 November 2019) has been observed to increase steadily and is predicted to continue, and some humans in isolated communities reaching extreme old age, with many people now living to mid-80 and beyond [2].

The two leading theories of ageing are the 'disposable soma theory' and the 'antagonistic pleiotropy theory' [3]. These theories are both evolutionary in nature and are attempts to explain why ageing takes place and why it may be necessary. The precise details of the theories are not relevant here but please refer to further reading. They both, essentially, say that physiologically we invest in the early and developmental stages of life with the aim of reproducing and that once our reproductive potential is past, we invest less physiologically in our bodies. This 'investment' is in the protective and regenerative functions of our body. As we age, we become less able to resist infection and to recover from injury. This has considerable face validity in the sense that as we age we become more frail, and with ageing the phenomenon of multipathology—whereby as people age, they tend to accumulate diseases—is more prominent.

2.3   The Underlying Processes that Lead to Ageing

It seems most likely that the biological processes that lead to ageing lie in our genes. Every structure—except the brain—in the body is continually being renewed and repaired. This takes place by the production of new cells, and these cells are produced in the process of mitosis whereby somatic cells divide to produce—in theory—two identical daughter cells. However, daughter cells are rarely identical to the cell from which they were derived and rarely identical to each other.

In the process of mitosis, the genetic material—the deoxyribonucleic acid (DNA)—contained in the chromosomes of the cell nucleus replicates. DNA is composed of 'base pairs'—pairs of molecules, which should always be the same in daughter cells and, largely, this is the case. However, the process of replication is not perfect, and we accumulate 'mutations' every time a cell divides [3], and a mutation is when the same base pair does not appear in a daughter cell as appeared in the original cell. Since base pairs—or sets of three base pairs called 'codons'—are the letters of the genetic code, this accumulation of errors eventually takes its toll. If cells accumulate ten mutations each time they divide, then after two divisions the subsequent daughter cell will have another ten mutations and so on over the lifespan and many thousands of cycles of mitosis [4]. The greater the accumulation of errors, the more different the daughter cells will become, and the more the structure and function of the body will be adversely affected until the total accumulation of errors is catastrophic for the body and it can no longer function. With ageing, the length of structures at the end of our chromosomes called telomeres reduces. This correlates with ageing, and in some progeroid syndromes whereby people age prematurely, the telomeres are shortened. The precise function of the telomeres is unknown, but it is possible that they have a protective function on the chromosomes and, thereby, the genetic material. One of the unavoidable causes of damage to our DNA is oxidative stress [5], which is due to our bodies having to survive in a relatively oxygen-rich environment. Of course, our bodies depend on oxygen, but it is in fact a very toxic substance. We perceive oxygen as being a positive component of life and, while this is true, is very reactive chemically and in reaction with, for example, the iron in haemoglobin, it can form a species of oxygen called 'superoxide', which is very toxic. However, our bodies have a range of mechanisms to protect us against oxygen toxicity. With age, these mechanisms become less efficient.

Nerve cells such as those in the brain do not undergo mitosis and, therefore, are protected from the accumulation of genetic errors. However, due to the lack of mitosis, nerve cells have a very limited capacity to regenerate, and damage to nerve cells is very hard to overcome. Other changes related to ageing, again take place in the brain such as the accumulation of unwanted proteins and areas of damage. Also, the brain is served by the cardiovascular system, and this is not protected from the accumulation of genetic errors, and there are other age-related changes in the cardiovascular system—to be considered below—which can have a deleterious effect on the brain.

Despite the theories of some researchers such as Aubrey de Grey of the SENS Research Foundation (https://www.sens.org/), it is unlikely that human beings can live indefinitely or even for periods extended beyond the currently recorded maximum lifespans, which, for some people, extend into the hundreds and even into double figures beyond that. But, as is often said by older people: 'old age does not come alone'. The writer Jonathan Swift presaged this in *Gulliver's Travels* when the subject of the book met the imaginary Struldbrugs who could never die. Swift recorded that, despite their immortality, they continued to age and became blind and bald and suffered other afflictions of ageing.

2.4 Cancer and Ageing

Cancer—while not confined to old age—is associated with ageing and is a result of the accumulation of genetic mutations in cells with ageing. The prevalence of cancer increases with ageing [6]. Cancer is also associated with risk factors such as smoking and exposure to sunlight, radiation, way of living and a range of harmful chemicals called 'carcinogens'. The combined effect of the accumulation of genetic mutations with age and the accumulated exposure to risk factors conspire to increase the risk of cancer, although cancer can arise in the absence of these risk factors. The body does try to defend itself against harmful cells using a process of 'surveillance', which finds and destroys cancer cells. But the combined accumulation of errors in old age and the decreasing ability of the body to defend itself against cancer cells leads to an increase in particular cancer types incidence with age [6].

2.5 Ageing of the Systems of the Body

I will now consider each of the systems of the body and how they are affected by ageing, and this is summarised in Table 2.1.

2.5.1 The Central Nervous System [6]

The central nervous system is comprised of the brain and the spinal cord. As already mentioned, the cells in this system are not replaced with ageing, and the cells in the system cannot regenerate; however, they do have some capacity to form new nerve connections to bypass damaged areas, for example, in stroke. Therefore, in one sense, it is protected against the effects of ageing seen in other systems as a result of the accumulation of errors during mitosis, and in fact, the brain and the central nervous system do not age like other systems. But they do age. In lay terms, with ageing the central nervous does 'slow down'. This effect is not dramatic, but the speed at which the nervous system works—the speed at which nerve impulses are transmitted—slows, and this is detectable when older people are tested and compared with younger people on reaction times. However, it should be emphasised that this effect is very small and unlikely to have much effect in everyday life. Sometimes, the effect of ageing on the brain is exaggerated, and many stereotypes exist regarding memory and personality. For example, it is commonly assumed that all older

Table 2.1 Summary of effects of ageing on the systems of the body

System	Effect
Central nervous system	Loss of nerve cells, reduced efficiency of nerve transmission, brain shrinks
Skin and hair	Skin: Loses fat layers and oil glands, wrinkling and loss of elasticity
	Hair loses pigmentation and turns grey
Cardiovascular	Atrophy of heart muscle, atherosclerosis
Respiratory	Loss of elasticity, rib cage atrophy
Skeletomuscular	Muscle: Atrophy and loss of tone and strength
	Bone: Loss of calcium, reduction in height, changes to joints
Digestive	Reduced acid and enzymes, reduced taste buds, reduced motility
Renal system	Reduced filtration capacity
Sensory	Eyes: Pupil size decreases, focusing takes longer, thickening of lens
	Ears: Decreased sensitivity to high frequencies, decreased pitch discrimination
	Taste: Reduced taste sensation, reduced smell
	Touch: Reduced sensitivity to heat cold and injury
Endocrine	Reduced metabolic rate, pituitary-hypothalamic axis less responsive
Reproductive	Desire and performance persist into seventh, eighth and ninth decades, atrophy of sexual organs and reduced vaginal fluids in females, reduced sperm production and enlarged prostate in men
Immune	Decreased ability to distinguish 'self' from 'non-self'

people have poor memories and that older people grow more stubborn with age. Nevertheless, memory is affected by ageing, and from approximately the 40 years old, the efficiency of our memories declines and continues into old age. This is not usually a problem for two reasons: the effect is usually small, and we have considerable reserve capacity in our brains; and as we age, we learn to compensate for declining memory. Younger people in their 20s may not need to keep a diary of upcoming events; someone in their 40s and beyond will almost certainly maintain one. On the other hand, confounding factors are at work, and we also become a great deal busier in our occupations and social lives as we age, at least up to the point of retirement. For some relatively young people, however, the loss of memory can interfere with everyday life and this is a syndrome known as age-associated memory impairment (AAMI). This is not severe, but it is persistent and a person with AAMI, while capable of functioning as in, for example, going shopping with the car may subsequently forget where the car has been parked. Of course, memory loss can become severe and incapacitating in dementia. It is not known if AAMI necessarily presages dementia and, in fact, if dementia is an inevitable aspect of ageing, but it is established that dementia is a condition of old age as the prevalence of dementia increases markedly with age. Dementia is a syndrome characterised by severe memory loss, amongst other things, and has several causes. The leading cause is Alzheimer's disease, followed by vascular dementia and Lewy body dementia. There are several other types of dementia, and it is possible to have more than one type of dementia, which is called mixed dementia. Alzheimer's disease is characterised by the presence of areas of devastation in the brain called plaques and tangles. The process usually originates in the hippocampus and then spreads to the lateral areas of the brain, especially affecting the temporal lobes and the cholinergic pathways. The brain volume of someone with Alzheimer's disease is significantly reduced. However, a definitive diagnosis of Alzheimer's disease can only be made post-mortem as biopsies of the brain are not done routinely. However, it should be noted that there are confounding cases regarding Alzheimer's disease whereby some people have vastly reduced brain volume and may even show evidence of plaques and tangles post-mortem without having shown any sign of cognitive decline in life. Nevertheless, these are rare cases. The underlying cause of Alzheimer's disease is not known and there is no cure; the process of cognitive decline cannot be reversed, and the use of drugs to restore the cholinergic pathways is minimal and short-term. Alzheimer's disease and other forms of dementia are not inevitable with old age, but it is associated with age. It is possible that if we all lived long enough, we may well all develop some form of dementia.

Regarding personality, it is known from longitudinal studies of ageing that personality is a stable construct; if we are born with a particular personality type, we take that personality type into old age and eventually we die with that personality type. It is worth noting that—in the absence of some form of dementia—intelligence does not reduce with age as demonstrated in longitudinal studies. Intelligence is composed of fluid and crystallised intelligence. Fluid intelligence is used to solve problems and crystallised intelligence is analogous to wisdom. It is known that fluid intelligence declines with age, but that overall intelligence does not. Therefore, with age we compensate for changes in fluid intelligence by using crystallised intelligence.

2.5.2 Skin [7]

The organ in which the process of ageing is most noticeable is the skin. This is because the skin covers the body and is visible, especially the face and hands. Likewise, the hair is visible, and the effects of ageing can be seen here too. The skin is a layered organ composed of tissues with proteins composed of elastin and collagen. We see the surface of the skin and the effects of ageing are noticeable here, but the skin is a layer of keratinised cells; it is dead, and the changes we notice are a result of changes in the layers beneath that. What we first notice about the ageing process in the skin is the development of wrinkles around the eyes and on the face generally. Then in later life, the skin starts to sag around the body. These changes are visible due to the main effect of ageing on the skin, which is a reduction in the protein elastin, and thereby a loss in the elasticity of the skin. This means that the skin does not hang as tightly around the body as we age, and it is easier to distort and slower to regain its initial form. The skin generally becomes thinner with age, and the combination of the ease with which the skin can be distorted and its thinning mean that the skin is more easily damaged as we age. The skin is also slower to repair in older age due to a less effective immune system, a reduced healing process and a lower blood supply to the skin. In addition to these changes, the layer of fat underneath the skin—the adipose layer—becomes thinner with age, and the insulating effect of the skin is reduced leading to a lower resistance to low temperatures.

2.5.3 Cardiovascular System [8]

The cardiovascular system is composed of the heart and the blood vessels, and it is adversely affected in ageing. It is important to understand that the cardiovascular system has considerable reserve capacity. In other words, healthy older people can adapt to the changes in the cardiovascular system, and the effects of ageing are only apparent if the system is challenged. For example, running to catch a bus will generally be harder for someone as they age, but going about the normal activities of daily life will not be affected. The effects of ageing on the cardiovascular system are threefold: loss of elasticity in the vessels of the system, the atherosclerotic changes in the walls of the arteries and the effects of ageing on the cardiac muscle. The loss of elasticity in the vessels of the cardiovascular system arise from ageing changes in the proteins that constitute the blood vessels. This loss of elasticity means that the system cannot adapt as rapidly as we age and, therefore, cannot accommodate changes in blood pressure as well as when we are younger. In the arteries, this is compounded by the atherosclerotic changes in the vessels whereby fatty deposits accumulate in the walls of the arteries, and calcium also accumulates making the walls of the arteries stiff. The heart is a muscle and all muscles age, but becoming atrophied and, thereby, weaker which means that blood is not circulated as efficiently with age, and the heart becomes less able to adapt to the changing needs of the body, especially when the blood circulation needs to be increased.

2.5.4 Respiratory System [9]

The respiratory system is affected by ageing by a reduction in both lung volume and lung elasticity. The latter arises due to a reduction in elastin in the structure of the lungs. In common with the cardiovascular system, the respiratory system has considerable reserve capacity, and we rarely call on all the capacity of the lungs as we carry out normal activities of living. However, if we challenge the capacity of the lungs, for example, in vigorous exercise, we observe the effects of ageing. Younger people have greater lung capacity than older people resulting from both the reduced elasticity and volume, and this affects all of the aspects of lung function. The principal effect is that the ability of the lungs to transfer atmospheric oxygen to the blood is reduced, and the concomitant ability to remove carbon dioxide from the blood to the atmosphere is reduced. Of course, the respiratory and cardiovascular system work together—sometimes referred to as the cardiorespiratory system—to oxygenate the blood, and it is very hard to consider one without considering the other.

2.5.5 Skeletomuscular System [10]

The skeletomuscular system is composed of the skeleton and the skeletal musculature, and both aspects are prone to the effects of ageing. The skeleton is composed of bone, and with age the bone tissue becomes less dense. This process is osteoporotic, and it takes place in both men and women, but only if it is causing a problem, for example, by bones collapsing or fracturing easily and even spontaneously (a pathological fracture) in someone identified as having the disease of osteoporosis. Other changes to take place in the skeleton affect the bones and the spinal cord, respectively. With age, the weight-bearing joints—knees and hips—accumulate damage, and articulation at these joints becomes less easy. This process is osteoarthritis—as distinct from rheumatoid arthritis (to be described later)—and can, in extreme cases, cause pain and immobility. It is a natural part of the ageing process, but not every older person is identified as having osteoarthritis. In the spinal cord, the cartilage, which separates and cushions the vertebrae, becomes thinner, and this can lead to a degree of deformity in the spinal cord known as kyphosis whereby the spinal cord curves outwards and the person develops an increasing stooped or 'hunched' posture. The thinning of these discs of cartilage decreases the distance between vertebrae and this leads to a loss in height. Again, these changes are quite normal, but for a few people can become problematic. The muscle tissue atrophies with age leading to a reduced muscle bulk and a progressively weaker musculature. This is not, in itself, problematic as the musculature, in common with many systems, has considerable reserve capacity but with age, combined with the effects of ageing on the cardiorespiratory system, the muscles become less efficient, especially if challenged as in extreme or unaccustomed exercise.

2.5.6 Digestive System [11]

A major component of the digestive system—running from the mouth to the anus—is smooth muscle, and like all the muscles of the body, this ages by atrophying. Nevertheless, the effects of ageing on the digestive system are quite minimal and often exaggerated. There may be a small propensity towards constipation with age as the smooth musculature weakens, but constipation is multifaceted, having other physiological and behavioural causes, so it is hard to isolate the effects of ageing on the smooth muscle of the digestive system. Changes in other systems such as the sensory system (affecting smell and taste) to be described below will also have an influence on the digestive system as older people's dietary habits may change. There is some evidence that the secretory and the absorptive functions of the digestive system reduce with age; again, this is likely to have a minimal effect under normal circumstances.

2.5.7 Renal System [12]

The renal system is composed of the kidneys and the urinary bladder. The main effect of ageing is on the kidneys, which reduce in volume and have less capacity to filter the blood. In normal health, this is not a problem but in disease, especially if the kidneys are affected, it can induce renal failure. Another consequence of reduced filtration with age is that many drugs are cleared from the blood less efficiently, and this can alter their therapeutic index whereby lower doses of some drugs may be required in older compared with younger people, and side effects and toxicity can develop at relatively lower doses.

2.5.8 Sensory System

It is conventional to consider the sensory system under the 'five senses' of sight, hearing, touch, taste and smell, and I will consider each of these in turn.

2.5.8.1 Sight [13]
It is very rare for sight not to be adversely affected by ageing. Wearing spectacles becomes increasingly common with old age, and this is mainly to correct long-sightedness, which develops as a result of changes in the shape of the lens in the eye. We also become less able to accommodate changes in light as a result of biochemical changes in the eye in the rods and cones, and with age the outer surface of the eye becomes increasingly opaque. This develops more quickly in some people who develop what are known as cataracts.

2.5.8.2 Hearing [13]
Another almost inevitable feature of ageing is a reduction in hearing. The range of sounds we can hear as we age reduces. The bones of the inner ear, which translate sound from the outer to the inner ear, become fused and less able to transmit that sound making hearing within the normal range of speech more difficult leading to some degree of deafness.

2.5.8.3 Touch
Sensitivity to touch declines with age, and this includes the senses of cold, heat and pain.

2.5.8.4 Taste and Smell
It is hard to separate taste and smell as the taste is largely dependent on our sense of smell. Both the sense of taste, on its own, and the sense of smell decline with age, and the effect of the decline in the sense of smell compounds the decline in the sense of taste.

2.5.9 Endocrine System [14]

In common with other systems, the endocrine system is affected by age, and this is manifested as a reduction in the extent to which the endocrine system responds to changes in the body. The link between the brain and the endocrine system is the hypothalamus pituitary axis, whereby changes sensed by the brain are passed on the pituitary system which, in turn, controls the endocrine system. This axis becomes less responsive with age, and one manifestation of this is the decreased ability to acclimatise as we age when we change time zones and move between regions of the world, where the temperature differs markedly.

2.5.10 Reproductive System [15]

Changes in the reproductive system are related to changes in the endocrine system, which release the sex hormones oestrogen and testosterone. These hormones are responsible, respectively, for the development of secondary sex characteristics in females and males and achieving reproductive potential. The levels of sex hormones in the body decline with age, and both sexes can report a reduction in libido. However, there is an abrupt change in the reproductive system in females, which mainly takes place between the ages of 40–50 called the menopause. The experience of the signs of menopause, principally hot flushes and changes to a cessation of monthly periods, varies between women, but ultimately ovulation ceases and reproductive potential ceases. In men, the effects of ageing on the reproductive system vary. The experience of the effect of ageing on the reproductive system in men also varies, but in men the effects are less severe and less abrupt. Loss of libido can occur and erectile dysfunction; however, men continue to produce sperm and maintain reproductive potential into old age.

2.5.11 Immune System [16]

The functions of the immune system reduce with age leading to an increased proneness to infection. The ability of the immune system to distinguish self from non-self also declines, and the incidence of auto-immunity—whereby the immune system can attack and destroy normal body tissues—increases. One common outcome of this is the disease known as rheumatoid arthritis. This is not a normal part of ageing but is more common with age.

2.6 Consequences of Physiological Ageing

Ageing is unpredictable in any individual, but the consequences for older people as a group are abundant. The distinction between the normal aspects of ageing and pathophysiological aspects of ageing is hard to define. Moreover, ageing itself is not a disease process, but for some people the combined effect of ageing on several systems can take a toll, and this can range from frailty—a general lowering in resilience to adversity and decreasing ability to carry out usual activities of daily living—to multipathology—where several pathological conditions coexist in one individual. The prevalence of both frailty and multipathology increases with old age, and one consequence of this is an increase in polypharmacy—the use of several drugs simultaneously [17]. Polypharmacy, in turn, brings its own problems with drug interactions and side effects. This is a particular problem in older people due to the reduced renal filtration referred to above, which necessitates reduced dosages of many drugs.

2.7   Mitigating the Effects of Ageing

Chronological ageing, of course, cannot be slowed, halted or reversed. It is also disputable how much the effects of ageing can be mitigated, but there are proposed markers of healthy biological ageing [18]. The evidence that the effects of ageing on the brain can be slowed down or dementia prevented, in vulnerable people, are mixed. Contrary to common misconceptions, the effects of ageing on the brain are not slowed down by using the brain, for example, by solving puzzles or engaging in intellectual activities. On the other hand, there is evidence that being physically active, especially throughout life, does have beneficial effects on the brain. In terms of the physical effects of ageing, exercise is definitely beneficial for the skeletomuscular and cardiorespiratory systems. Briefly, weight-bearing exercise is beneficial for the skeleton as it helps to prevent osteoporosis and likewise helps to maintain muscle mass and muscle strength. Likewise, exercise for older people can improve cardiac output and respiratory function. Clearly, it is better to enter old age fit, but it is also clear that taking up exercise in old age is beneficial; it is never too late.

2.8   Summary

That the body ages physiologically is indisputable. Why the body ages physiologically is unknown, and how the body ages is only dimly understood. While the answer to the causes of ageing possibly lies largely in our genes, there is probably a combination of factors causing the body to age physiologically.

2.9   Suggested Further Reading and URLs

Theories of ageing are reviewed in this excellent article by Kunlin Jin (2010) titled 'Modern biological theories of aging' published in Ageing and Disease: https://www.ncbi.nlm.nih.gov/pmc/articles/PMC2995895/

Aubrey de Grey believes that ageing can be halted, allowing people to live forever. It is worth listening to this charismatic and effective public speaker, whether or not you agree with him. George Williams (see Antagonistic Pleiotropy Theory of Aging below) believes that anti-ageing research is a fundamentally foolish endeavour, a 'chase after the fountain of youth'. https://www.ted.com/talks/aubrey_de_grey_says_we_can_avoid_aging

Ageing is not necessarily accompanied by disease, but some diseases are more common with and appear to be related to ageing and they are reviewed here: https://www.age.mpg.de/healthy-ageing/age-related-diseases/dementia/

Baltimore Longitudinal Study of Aging. One of the longest established studies of ageing; access requires registration here: https://www.blsa.nih.gov/

Can Science extend lifespan and improve the quality of late-life health? Dr. Jennifer Tullet, Biosciences lecturer and researcher at the University of Kent, discusses current research into the ageing process (mostly about worms, but very interesting). https://www.youtube.com/watch?v=qRn5hHJi_Ds

The Lothian Birth Cohort of 1921 and 1936. These longitudinal studies of ageing are amongst the most definitive on the effects of ageing on cognitive function, physical function and health, and the complete list of publications can be accessed here: https://www.lothianbirthcohort.ed.ac.uk/

References

1. McDonald RB (2014) Biology of ageing. Garland Science, New York
2. Edwards EA (1973) Extreme old age. JAMA 225(4):419–419
3. Kirkwood TBL (2011) Systems biology of ageing and longevity. Phil. Trans. R. Soc. B. 366:64–70
4. Partridge L (2010) The new biology of ageing. Phil Trans R Soc B 365:147–154
5. Finkel T, Holbrook NJ (2000) Oxidants, oxidative stress and the biology of ageing. Nature 408:239–247
6. de Magalhães J (2013) How ageing processes influence cancer. Nat Rev Cancer 13:357–365
7. Nigam Y, Knight J (2017a) Anatomy and physiology of ageing 11: the skin. Nurs Times 113(12):51–55. https://www.nursingtimes.net/roles/older-people-nurses-roles/anatomy-and-physiology-of-ageing-11-the-skin-27-11-2017/. Accessed 6 Sept 2019
8. Knight J, Nigam Y (2017b) Anatomy and physiology of ageing 1: the cardiovascular system. Nurs Times 113(2):22–24. https://www.nursingtimes.net/roles/older-people-nurses-roles/anatomy-and-physiology-of-ageing-1-the-cardiovascular-system-31-01-2017/. Accessed 6 Sept 2019
9. Knight J, Nigam Y (2017c) Anatomy and physiology of ageing 2: the respiratory system. Nurs Times 113(3):53–55. https://www.nursingtimes.net/roles/older-people-nurses-roles/anatomy-and-physiology-of-ageing-2-the-respiratory-system-2-27-02-2017/. Accessed 6 Sept 2019
10. Knight J, Nigam Y, Hore N (2017a) Anatomy and physiology of ageing 10: the musculoskeletal system. Nurs Times 113(11):60–63. https://www.nursingtimes.net/roles/older-people-nurses-roles/anatomy-and-physiology-of-ageing-10-the-musculoskeletal-system-30-10-2017/. Accessed 6 Sept 2019
11. Nigam Y, Knight J (2017b) Anatomy and physiology of ageing 3: the digestive system. Nurs Times 113(4):54–57. https://www.nursingtimes.net/roles/older-people-nurses-roles/anatomy-and-physiology-of-ageing-3-the-digestive-system-27-03-2017/. Accessed 6 Sept 2019
12. Andrade M, Knight J (2017) Anatomy and physiology of ageing 4: the renal system. Nurs Times 113(5):46–49. https://www.nursingtimes.net/roles/older-people-nurses-roles/anatomy-and-physiology-of-ageing-4-the-renal-system-02-05-2017/. Accessed 6 Sept 2019
13. Knight J, Wigham C, Nigam Y (2017b) Anatomy and physiology of ageing 6: the eyes and ears. Nurs Times 113(7):39–42. https://www.nursingtimes.net/roles/older-people-nurses-roles/anatomy-and-physiology-of-ageing-6-the-eyes-and-ears-26-06-2017/. Accessed 6 Sept 2019
14. Knight J, Nigam Y (2017d) Anatomy and physiology of ageing 7: the endocrine system. Nurs Times 113(8):48–51. https://www.nursingtimes.net/roles/older-people-nurses-roles/anatomy-and-physiology-of-ageing-7-the-endocrine-system-31-07-2017/. Accessed 6 Sept 2019
15. Knight J, Nigam Y (2017e) Anatomy and physiology of ageing 8: the reproductive system. Nurs Times 113(9):44–47. https://www.nursingtimes.net/roles/older-people-nurses-roles/anatomy-and-physiology-of-ageing-8-the-reproductive-system-29-08-2017/. Accessed 6 Sept 2019

16. Nigam Y, Knight J (2017c) Anatomy and physiology of ageing 9: the immune system. Nurs Times 113(10):42–45. https://www.nursingtimes.net/roles/older-people-nurses-roles/anatomy-and-physiology-of-ageing-9-the-immune-system-21-09-2017/. Accessed 6 Sept 2019
17. Cantlay A, Glynn T, Barton N (2016) Polypharmacy in the elderly. InnovAiT 9(2):69–77
18. Mathers JC, Deary IJ, Kuh D, Lord JM, Khaw K-T, Lara J, Nussan J, Cooper R, Ginty A (2012) Guidelines for biomarkers of healthy ageing. Medical Research Council, London

Life History of Older People: Social Theories and the Sociology of Ageing

3

Susan Thornton

Contents

3.1 Learning Objectives

This chapter will provide you with the knowledge to:

- Identify how ideas from the sociology of ageing can "shape" an individual's experience of growing old
- Examine the importance of narrative and biography to personal well-being
- Reflect upon ways in which a "life history" approach can enhance the care of the older person in a range of health and social care environments

3.2 Introduction

Ageing is a multifaceted and complex phenomenon with biological, psychosocial, cultural and spiritual factors playing a vital role in determining why and how we grow old. As Phillips et al. observe [1], each facet of ageing is intimately and

S. Thornton (✉)
Department of Nursing, School of Health and Social Care, Centre of Excellence in Healthcare Education, Staffordshire University, Shrewsbury, UK

© Springer Nature Switzerland AG 2021
W. McSherry et al. (eds.), *Understanding Ageing for Nurses and Therapists*,
Perspectives in Nursing Management and Care for Older Adults,
https://doi.org/10.1007/978-3-030-40075-0_3

inextricably related: biological senescence (the physical process of ageing) both determines and is determined by our psychological, spiritual and social well-being.

This chapter focuses explicitly upon the sociological dimension of ageing, ways in which society can influence our attitudes towards older people and, therefore, from a health and social care perspective, helps to define the quality of care which they receive. It will draw upon ideas from the general discipline of sociology and social gerontology, a subset of gerontology (the study of ageing), which has enjoyed a recent surge in popularity amongst the health and social care research community [1–3]. The nature and importance of life history or life story/biographical approaches, as imbedded in and evolving from sociological discourse, will also be explored.

Throughout the chapter, readers are encouraged to reflect upon and explore the application of ideas within their own care settings through practice examples and reflective activities. This will offer an opportunity to examine personal views about age and ageing, which are central to effectively meeting the care needs of older people in a variety of care environments.

3.3 Social Theories of Age and Ageing: An Introductory Overview

There are many distinct ways of viewing and explaining society. Which theoretical position is adopted will depend upon a sociologist's preferred perspective or underpinning value position about how the social world works [4]. As theoretical standpoints are numerous and complex, an attempt has been made to simplify and categorise some of the main themes which have emerged and highlight their relevance to working with older people in the health and social care sectors. In particular, there is focus upon a number of key ideas, which underpin and inform life history approaches.

3.3.1 Traditional Approaches

Theories of society can be broadly distinguished between those that propose "top down" or "bottom up" explanations about society, which in turn will influence how society is investigated and recommendations for promoting social well-being. "Top down" theories offer what is sometimes referred to as macro or structural perspectives [4]. These are concerned with the way in which the different parts or foundations, which make up the fabric of society, fit together and interact. For example, what role do institutions such as the economy, politics, religion, education and healthcare play in influencing when a person is defined as old and their existential journey through the later stages of the life course. Conversely, "Bottom up" or micro, social action perspectives highlight the experiences and choices which we make, our individual "agency", throughout our lives. This will in turn impact upon our own attitudes towards meanings and expectations of old age with individuals rather than society controlling how old age is viewed and experienced [4].

Another dilemma which concerns sociologists is that of consensus versus conflict. Do societies exist in harmony and order through shared goals, values and beliefs systems or are they characterised by division and inequality [1, 4]? Both premises have many potential applications to healthcare and the social position of older people. For example, as people grow older, do they tend to "disengage" from their normal social roles and contacts including employment: a mutually beneficial transaction between the older person and society, which enables the transfer of power from the old to the young, and thus the continuing stability of a natural (evolutionary) social order? Or does society (and the older individual themselves) benefit from our seniors remaining active and involved in old age, either adopting new roles and social identities or continuing with the lifestyles beliefs and behaviours, which they have acquired earlier in their life course [4]? Each of these approaches emphasises the need to maintain a harmonious and stable society, although have differing views about the ways in which the older generation can contribute to this goal.

Conversely, conflict theorists working within the wider remit of critical sociology focus upon inequality, imbalances in power relationships and the way in which structural factors, including wealth and privilege serve to oppress and disadvantage certain social groups such as the old and frail [3, 4]. There are many variants on this theme, for example, attributing the loss of power and influence in old age to the growth of industrialisation and modernisation or demonstrating how a person's status and prestige are dictated by the age group or strata to which they belong, thus determining access to social opportunity and resources. This includes investigations into the way in which specific social institutions such as a county's welfare system including nationalised healthcare systems, may construct dependency and disempowerment in old age, rather than helping their older clientele [5].

3.3.2 Contemporary Approaches

Some of the more contemporary sociological approaches to explaining ageing adopt a much more nuanced and individualistic standpoint, focusing upon micro-level interactions which occur and define our own personal experiences of ageing. An example of this is Lars Tornstam's developmental theory of gerotranscendence, which proposes that as we become older we tend to move beyond the rather limited narrow views of life associated with our younger years, becoming less self-centred and more focused upon things that are meaningful to us and that we enjoy [6]. This involves recalling and re-examining the lives we have lived and the choices we have made. The ability to reminisce and place meaningful interpretations on past life is of vital relevance to the notion of life history and will be expanded upon in a subsequent section.

The therapeutic benefits and enhanced life satisfaction associated with the process of gerotranscendence have been widely documented. These include greater life satisfaction, increased resiliency in retirement, enhanced motivation and the promotion of physical and mental well-being [6]. In addition, as Rajani and Jarwaid [6] observe, Tornstam's theory is interesting because, as a natural process, it has universal applicability across continents, cultures and care settings. From a caring perspective, it potentially provides nurses and other health and social care practitioners with a useful frame of reference to promote positive attitudes towards growing old.

3.4   Ageism, Stigma and Stereotyping

Social attitudes towards ageing and the nature and persistence of social stereotypes are a key concern for social gerontologists. Prejudice and oppression may occur at any stage of the life course although much attention has been focused upon the impact of these processes upon older people and the often deleterious outcomes for their well-being [7–9]. Ageism refers to treating people differently and generally less favourably because of their age and arises from prejudices and intolerant beliefs systems, which often have their basis in damaging and inappropriate stereotypes. The latter refers to a set of fixed and overgeneralised ideas that are held about people or social groups. Negative stereotypes generate a fear of difference, people who are perceived as not "like us" or "the other", and involve a process of labelling individuals with social characteristics, which is viewed as unacceptable and undesirable. This results in stigma, which may be "felt" by the individual as a mark of shame and disgrace and "enacted" by other members of society through discriminatory and exclusionary behaviours [10].

Ageism directed against older people is perceived as having its basis in a set of "myths" or misconceptions about the abilities and social value of our elders. Older people may internalise these values, thereby reinforcing and perpetuating the stereotypical assumptions that are held by the wider members of their community [7, 10]. Conventionally, Western societies are regarded as more ageist than Eastern societies, focusing upon decline and physical, cognitive and financial ineptitude rather than the spiritual growth and acquired wisdom of advancing years. Yet, both these views have been subject to challenge citing the pervasive presence of ageism across all cultural boundaries and the availability of social and economic resources being the most influential factor in determining attitudes towards our older citizens [11]. Moreover, older people may not merely experience discrimination on the basis of age but are often subject to multiple oppression, relating to the intersection of other categories of social such as race, ethnicity and gender, which may lead to significant poverty, ill health, housing disadvantage and social isolation, creating a "double" or even "triple jeopardy" of social discrimination [12].

3.4.1   Impact of Ageism

The potential scope and consequences of ageism are far-reaching. In the context of health and social care, beliefs and misconceptions are often deep-rooted and resistant to change, serving to undermine the quality of care provided and appear to persist across a wide range of international healthcare systems [9]. Such ageist assumptions are frequently implicit and expressed through unconscious bias rather than explicit actions and behaviours, therefore, potentially becoming an inherent feature of everyday practice [13].

Developing awareness of our hidden and sometimes institutionally entrenched prejudices and beliefs about ageing is essential for healthcare practitioners to ensure that we remain non-judgemental and deliver the highest quality of care possible. In response to this, a number of initiatives have been developed to counteract ageism amongst healthcare workers, with some excellent examples of high-quality practice both locally and internationally [14, 15].

There is increasing emphasis placed throughout the international literature on the importance of successful and active ageing [2]. Both these concepts attempt to countermand conventional negative stereotypes of older people with a more positive image of the social value and contributions that can be made in later life, stressing the importance of exploiting talents, experience and skills gained over the life course to promote a healthy and productive old age. However, such approaches have also been subject to rigorous criticism, accused of privileging the "young old" over the "frail old" [2, 3]. This has the effect of devaluing the experience of older people who by virtue of comorbidities and dependency may be unable to meet the criterion set by the "happy gerontology" paradigm [3, p. 93] but may equally regard their lives as rewarding and worthwhile [2].

On a micro-interactional level, other commentators have focused upon the benefits of promoting intergenerational relationships in combating ageist beliefs and misconceptions and sharing generational activity within intergenerational contact initiatives [14, 15]. Intergroup contact may be employed in several ways, for example, via family relationships, friendships, social and healthcare contact and every day interactions [14]. Alleged benefits include a reduction in negative attitudes towards older people and damaging age stereotypes, thus helping to counteract both direct and indirect ageism, providing opportunities for forging friendships and closer intergenerational ties [14].

The following practice example demonstrates how an intragenerational approach can be implemented within a health and social care setting.

Practice Example: The Role of Intergenerational Playgroups in Aged Care
Maria is an activity and lifestyle therapist in a residential care facility for aged residents with mild to moderate cognitive impairment. She has recently become concerned about a lack of interaction between residents and an apparent apathy to join in with some of the social activities. However, Maria has noticed that some of the older people seem to become notably more animated and actively engaged in their surroundings, in the company of children who often accompany visiting family members.

Maria raises this issue at the weekly staff meeting. Johan, one of the registered nursing practitioners, says that he has recently read an article about the benefits of intragenerational playgroup and wonders if it might be possible to introduce a similar scheme in their own establishment. Following discussion with the care managers and ensuring that legal and professional guidelines for safe practice are in place, Maria devises a diversional therapy/lifestyle programme, which facilitates interaction between three generations: the older residents, child carers (parent's relatives and nannies) and preschool children. This comprises a weekly 2 h session facilitated by a diversional therapist and involving participation in and variety of shared activities including singing, baking, painting and structured and unstructured play. A month's trial period is commenced.

Feedback suggests that everyone has benefited from this activity, increasing awareness and understanding of the needs of different age groups. For the older people, it seems to have provided them with a new zest for life, allowing them to make new friends, giving them a more clearly defined sense of roles and purpose and increasing their sense of dignity.

3.4.2 The Impact of Language

One interesting dimension of social interaction which makes a significant contribution towards what we believe and, therefore, how we behave is the role of language. This has led to a theoretical conundrum known as the Sapir-Whorf hypothesis. Put simply, does language determine thought or does thought determine language [16]? The power of words is undeniable. When we refer to the "miserable old man", the "sweet little old lady" or even "the elderly", we are reflecting not only ageist, but powerful gender stereotypes making automatic and damaging assumptions about person's roles, intentions and capabilities. We are also at risk of devaluing individuality and personhood through the process of homogenisation (allocating all older people to one social category) and infantilisation (treating older people as children), and therefore, incapable of choice, control and self-determination [10].

In health and social care, comments are often made using powerful language to describe the global demographic shifts in age structure such as the "greying" of the population or the "Silver Tsunami" and the perceived increased burden, which this places on healthcare resources. Jenny Bristow [17] has referred to this emotive and homogenising choice of words as "Doomography", claiming it is indicative of a wider gerontophobia, the idea that the increasing numbers of elderly population are a threat to the well-being of the wider population.

Reflective Question 1
Can changing the words which we use alter our views of older people?
Reflect upon the terms and expressions which you use to describe older people within your own workplace.

- *Do they generate positive or negative images of growing old?*
- *Does this have an impact upon the way that older people are treated?*
- *Will changing the language and terminology have a direct impact upon the quality of care that we can provide for older people and their carers?*

Just as language can play an important role in determining how we think about older people, it also forms a vital medium in enabling older people to communicate their life stories, hopes, dreams and aspirations: how they were, are and want to be viewed as a person, helping us to challenge our biases and stereotypical assumptions. The following section considers how the power of narrative, past and present can be employed as a therapeutic tool to promote compassionate person-centred care.

3.5 Life History Approaches: Introduction and Origins

Growing old should not be viewed as a singular event but a natural continuation of the life course and the culmination of previous life experiences [7]. There are many different dimensions of our existence, which make us the unique person we are today, family, work, leisure, loves, hates and fears. A person's present is inextricably linked to their past. Life history approaches empower older people to communicate the stories of their lives, linking past to present and enabling us as carers, to see the person beyond the diagnosis [18].

Life history methods were initially pioneered by anthropologists and later adopted by sociologists in an effort to better understand the life experiences of specific social groups, for example, native American Indians and other indigenous communities [4]. This was later adapted and applied to the healthcare arena by social scientists of symbolic interactionist tradition, such as Erving Goffman in his landmark studies of the experience of mental illness within institutional settings [19]. The importance and practical relevance of the approach has enjoyed a popular revival within contemporary gerontological nursing literature and regarded as fundamental to the ethos of delivering person-centred care [20].

3.5.1 Explaining Life Story Work

Essentially, life history, also referred to as biography or life story work, is used as a practical intervention with the aim of promoting person-centred care [18]. In relation to preferred terminology, most contemporary authorities tend to adopt the expression, "life story work", perhaps to distinguish this very specific application from broader methodological approaches within the social sciences. Therefore, this will also be the preferred term for the remainder of the chapter.

As we have noted in the previous sections, damaging stereotypes about older people often operate by way of generalisation, based upon the premise that all older people share common, often negative characteristics, which do not allow for variation and individuality. For health and social care practitioners, this may create a barrier in our ability to provide holistic person-centred care. Life story work helps us to visualise life from the perspective of the storyteller [20]. This assists us in countering our misconceptions about ageing, providing a framework which we can utilise to understand the uniqueness of our older patients and clients, and ensuring that the care needs of both themselves and their family and/or carers are central to the care planning process [21]. The "taking it further" example at the end of this section provides a specific account of some of the way in which narratives provided by older people can enable a clearer insight into their world in addition to improving cognitive and physical function.

Life story approaches are particularly pertinent to the area of dementia care, where older people are often unable to communicate specific characteristics of their identity. Tom Kitwood's seminal work on the need to preserve personhood of people with dementia through the implementation of person-centred care highlights the importance of biography in helping to restore self-esteem and social identity [22]. Additionally, understanding and validating what often appear to be challenging or irrational behaviours from the perspective of the person with dementia is of vital importance. Adopting a life history approach enables a "Deep Dive" into an older person's past which in turn assists in rationalising their present, thus supporting the implementation of appropriate strategies and techniques to de-escalate traumatic events [18, 23].

> **Reflective Question 2**
> *Think about what is important to you about your life making brief notes on the following:*
>
> *What do you value?*
> - *Who do you value?*
> - *What are the things in life that contribute to your sense of self?*
> - *What are the things that make you who you are/are part of your identity?*
>
> *Imagine you were put in a situation where you were unable to communicate these important personal characteristics to the people around you.*
>
> - *How would you feel? How might this impact upon your own and other people's perceptions of your social value?*
> - *Which of the things you think that define you, as an individual person, do you consider the most important?*

All the factors identified above are what helps to establish our status as a person determining our individual needs and aspirations. Denying or ignoring these elements of being can result in a process of social devaluation leading to a lack of agency and social esteem. Knowing and respecting a person's unique biography can restore help to make them feel valued with an important role to play in their future care and well-being.

3.5.2 Life Story Work: Benefits and Applications

The alleged benefits of life story work have been widely documented throughout the literature (i.e. [18, 20, 21, 23]). Common themes focus upon the restoration of personhood, increased collaboration and partnership and enhance the ability to make cognitive, interpersonal and practical connections. From the perspective of the older person, accessing memories of significant events and past achievements is perceived as fostering a sense of pride, restoring dignity and self-esteem and building resilience [18, 21]. Active participation within the care process can create a sense of ownership and agency, determining what information is disclosed and how this might be used to inform their future care. Moreover, the advantages associated with the process of reminiscence are perhaps not merely confined to aspects of mental well-being. Reflecting upon one's past may also result in physical improvements in mobility, for example, demonstrating balance, movement and actions that an older person may have used at a former point in their life course [24].

It is claimed that family members may also benefit through an increased sense of purpose, greater clarity of their roles within the caring relationship and the ability to view their loved one in a different and often more positive way [18, 21]. For care practitioners, engagement in life story work enables them to "See the person" beyond the diagnosis, thus placing them in a better position to identify and meet the older person's unique care needs.

However, life story work is not without its critics. Some commentators [18, 21, 25] advise caution when implementing this approach as remembering past events can sometimes be distressing perhaps evoking painful memories and reminders of unreconciled loss. This is particularly the case for older people with memory problems, so life history methods need to be applied sensitively and judiciously [21]. Time constraints and lack of experience, knowledge and confidence on the part of the healthcare professional are other potential barriers which need to be recognised and addressed [18, 21]. Consequently, several authorities such as Grøndahl et al. [25] contend that the research base for unequivocally establishing the benefits of life story work is limited, and much more rigorous investigation is required to fully assess the impact of this popular and widespread intervention.

3.5.3 Implementing Life Story Work: Formats, Tools and Processes

As Thompson [21] observes, careful planning when introducing life story work is essential. This raises several key considerations, which can be summarised as follows:

- **What** information is required?
- **How** is this obtained and stored?
- **Why** is it needed?

Information gathering will focus upon the collection of personal biographical details relating to the older person's past, present and future preferences capturing and storing those precious memories that they have acquired on their journey through the life course [25]. Likes and dislikes, hobbies, interests and the idiosyncrasies of everyday living can be captured and recorded to create an image of the older person as they want to be seen, not merely through the distorting prism of age, ill health or some other convenient social label. Capturing personal highlights, achievements and successes are also vital in instilling a sense of pride and restoring self-esteem, which might have been eroded by health problems, decreasing mental capacity and increasing physical dependency [21].

When implementing a life story approach, the importance of time, privacy and the actual pacing of activity is a prime consideration [18]. Obtaining information in short bursts may be preferable to lengthy formal interviews, both for the older person and their relatives. The wishes of the older person and the need to maintain confidentiality should always be paramount. Also, the purpose for implementing a life story approach needs to be made clear and agreed by all concerned, and if the older person chooses to decline, then this must be respected [21].

As Kindell et al. [23] note, many formats can be utilised for implementing life story work including life story books, collages, DVDs and reminiscence or memory boxes. Profile documents, which provide a summary of the older person's personal narrative, are relatively easy to compile and, therefore, have utility within busy acute care environments. A variety of free templates may be accessed via the Internet underpinning research (see further reading for links to these resources).

Hard copy life story resources are undoubtedly useful in terms of their tangible tactile properties. Touching a photograph of a loved one, holding a personal mementoes or keepsake from one's past can evoke a range of emotions and memories both happy and sad, engaging a range of sensory reactions, which has been demonstrated to have been of particular benefit in reminiscence work [25]. With the growth of technology and digital resources, social network platforms and apps can also be exploited to great advantage as a means of capturing, storing and updating life story material [21]. Indeed, there are several commercial apps available, which enable an older person to curate precious memories by uploading photographs, together with an audio message. Websites such as Dementia UK provide a summary of some of the more popular online resources: see further reading for links.

It is recognised, however, that not all older people will be comfortable, conversant with, or have the skills, motivation or mental capacity required to use digital resources. Access and affordability to digital devices may also be a potential barrier [21]. Nevertheless, the increasing importance and usage of technology in all its forms as an adjunct to more conventional methods of life story work will perhaps gain in popularity for forthcoming generations, and therefore, as healthcare workers, we should be aware of this potential.

Direct involvement of the older person and, where relevant, significant others such as family members and carers is vital to the success of implementing life history work, enabling ownership and empowerment. Thus, the relationship between the care professional and their patients or clients should be one of inclusivity, mutual support and collaboration rather than clinical expert and passive recipient [18]. This includes consulting the older person from the outset, encouraging them to make decisions in relation to purpose, method and intended outcomes of the life story enterprise. It is their story, after all which should act as the main impetus for care, as demonstrated in the following case example.

3.5.4   Taking It Further

Older Person's Narrations on Falls and Falling: Stories of Courage and Endurance

Clancy et al. [24] conducted a study in the north of Norway, which explored the perceptions of older people in five care facilities regarding falls, falling and falls prevention. A narrative approach was adopted, which enabled the older people to articulate their own accounts, perspectives and priorities based upon their own personal experiences. The intention of the study was to utilise the older person's perceptions to inform and contextualise future falls prevention and health promotion strategies.

The study found that the actual experience of a fall, which had been prioritised by the researchers as the most significant event, was accorded less of a priority by the older people. They did not want to dwell upon the implications and consequences of falling, but what was important was the opportunity to tell stories about their former lives, strength and endurance. Telling these tales of times past brought them to life, thus establishing a sense of purpose and control.

The authors describe this transformative process as a "form of mental time travel" (p. 7) recalling memories of strength, vitality and well-being. To illustrate the beneficial results associated with reminiscence about times past, they provide an example of a highly dependent resident who was normally immobilised by severe pain but became a "multitasking genius" when given the opportunity to narrate about his life. Story telling seemed to overcome the stigma and embarrassment associated with falling, prompting the residents to recall what they could do rather than their disabilities. Reminders of their former abilities restored appeared to validate the older people's sense of identity, self-esteem and social value.

The study is also instructive in that it demonstrates what was of actual importance to the older people concerned, rather than what we as the health and social care experts deem to be the priority.

- *Focusing upon your own area of practice, try to identify examples of specific occasions when there has been a difference in the care priorities identified by health and social care practitioners and the older people for whom you are caring.*
- *Explore ways in which life story work may help to overcome these mismatches in expectation about the purpose and outcomes of care.*

3.6   Summary of Main Points

The concept of person-centred care is of crucial importance in promoting the physical and psychosocial well-being of older people, restoring their sense of purpose, identity and social esteem. Life history or life story methods can assist care practitioners in facilitating a person-centred approach.

This chapter has attempted to focus upon several social factors, which will assist health and social care practitioners to develop the knowledge and skills required to implement life story techniques. This includes providing an overview of some of the key ideas underpinning the sociology of ageing including examples of traditional and contemporary sociological approaches to explaining ageing, the nature and impact of age discrimination and the power of language. The nature, potential benefits and challenges of life story work have also been highlighted together with practical suggestions for ways in which this might be implemented.

3.7   Suggested Reading

1. Giddens A, and Sutton P W. *Essential Concepts in Sociology.*2nd edition, Polity Press; 2017.This provides a general sociology textbook which is written in an interesting and accessible way provides an engaging introduction to sociology.
2. Sociology of Ageing Handbook. https://link.springer.com/book/10.1007/978-1-4419-7374-0 https://epdf.pub/queue/handbook-of-sociology-of-aging.html. This compromises 45 chapters written by world renown authors and will allow you to explore in much more detail all of the key themes highlighted in this introductory chapter.
3. Dementia UK www.Dementiauk.org
   https://www.dementiauk.org/for-professionals/free-resources/life-story-work/?gclid=EAIaIQobChMI1fPLqaqr5gIVVYjVCh3w5wqpEAAYASAAEgLYdvD_BwE
   An extremely useful and accessible website which offers a range of free life story work tools and templates for use by both lay people and health and social care professionals. Also provides practical tips and advice to guide implementation.
4. Drury L, Abrams D, Swift HJ. Making intergenerational Connections- an Evidence Review. Age UK, London: 2017.
   https://www.ageuk.org.uk/globalassets/age-uk/documents/reports-and--publications/reports-and-briefings/active-communities/rb_2017_making_intergenerational_connections.pdf
   interesting report that pulls together the evidence about the nature and value of intergenerational initiatives suggests ways in which these can be implemented. These principles which may be of value within the health and social care sector

References

1. Phillips JE, Ajrouch KJ, Hillcoat-Nalletamby S (2010) Key concepts in social gerontology. Sage, Boston
2. Katz S, Calasanti T (2015) Critical perspectives on successful ageing: does it "appeal more than it illuminates"? Gerontologist 55(1):26–33
3. Van Dyke S (2014) The appraisal of difference: critical gerontology and the active-ageing-paradigm. J Aging Stud 31:93–103
4. Giddens A, Sutton PW (2017) Essential concepts in sociology, 2nd edn. Polity Press, Cambridge

5. Yuill C, Crinson I, Duncan E (2010) Key concepts in health studies. Sage, Boston
6. Rajani F, Jawaid H (2015) Theory of gerotranscendence: an analysis. Aust J Psychiatr Behav Sci 2(1):1035. https://www.austinpublishinggroup.com/psychiatry-behavioral-sciences/full-text/ajpbs-v2- id1035.php. Accessed 3 Dec 2019
7. Ayalon L, Tech-Römer C (2018) Contemporary perspectives on ageism. International perspectives on ageing, vol 19. Springer, Cham, pp 1–11. https://link.springer.com/content/pdf/10.1007%2F978-3-319-73820-8.pdf. Accessed 3 Dec 2019
8. Bratt C, Abrams D, Swift HJ, Vauclair C-M, Marques S (2018) Perceived age discrimination across age in Europe: from an ageing society to a society for all ages. Dev Psychol 54(1):167–180
9. Wyman F, Shiovitz-Ezra S, Bengel J (2018) Ageism in the healthcare system. Providers, patient and systems. In: Ayalon L, Tech-Römer C (eds) Contemporary perspectives on ageism. International perspectives on ageing, vol 19. Springer, Cham, pp 193–212. https://link.springer.com/content/pdf/10.1007%2F978-3-319-73820-8.pdf. Accessed 3 Dec 2019
10. Voss P, Bodner E, Rothermund K (2018) Ageism: the relationship between age stereotype and age discrimination. In: Ayalon L, Tech-Römer C (eds) Contemporary perspectives on ageism. International perspectives on ageing, vol 19. Springer, Cham, pp 193–212. https://link.springer.com/content/pdf/10.1007%2F978-3-319-73820-8.pdf. Accessed 3 Dec 2019
11. Marquet M, Missotten P, Schroyen S, Nindaba D, Adam S (2016) Ageism in Belgium and Burundi: a comparative analysis. Clin Interv Ageing 11:1129–1139
12. De Noronha N (2019) Housing and older ethnic minority population in England. Race Equality Foundation, London
13. Gendron TL, Welleford AE, Inker J, White JT (2016) The language of ageism: why we need to use words carefully. The Gerontologist 56(6):997–1006
14. Drury L, Abrams D, Swift HJ (2017) Making intergenerational connections-an evidence review. Age UK, London
15. Gerritzen EV, Hull MJ, Verbeek H, Smith AE, Boer D (2020) Successful elements of intergenerational dementia programs: a scoping review. J Intergenerational Relationships 18:214–245. https://www.tandfonline.com/doi/full/10.1080/15350770.2019.1670770. Accessed 9 Dec 2019
16. Perlovosky L (2009) Language and emotions: emotional Sapir-Whorf hypothesis. Neural Netw 22:518–526
17. Bristow J (2019) Baby boomers and the pensions crisis: Doomography and Gerontophobia. Institute and Faculty of Actuaries, London
18. McKinney A (2017) The value of life story work for staff, people with dementia and family members. Nurs Older People 29(5):25–29
19. Shalin DN (2013) Goffman on mental illness: asylums and "the insanity of place" revisited. Symb Interact 37(1):122–144
20. Jefferies D, Hatcher D (2018) Developing person-centred care through the biographies of the older adult. J Nurs Educ 57(12):742–746
21. Thompson R (2011) Using life story work to enhance care. Nurs Older People 23(8):16–21
22. Kitwood T (1997) Dementia reconsidered: the person comes first. Open University Press, Buckingham
23. Kindell J, Burrows S, Wilkinson R, Keady JD (2014) Life story resources in dementia care. A review. Qual Ageing Older Adults 15(3):151–161
24. Clancy A, Balteskard B, Perander B, Mahler M (2015) Older persons 'narrations on falls and falling-Stories of courage and endurance. Int J Qual Stud Health Wellbeing 10:26123. https://www.ncbi.nlm.nih.gov/pmc/articles/PMC4288919/pdf/QHW-10-26123.pdf. Accessed 9 Dec 2019
25. Grøndahl VA, Persenius M, Bååth C, Helgeson AK (2017) The use of life stories and its influence on persons with dementia and their relatives and staff-a systematic mixed studies review. BMC Nurs 16:28. https://www.ncbi.nlm.nih.gov/pmc/articles/PMC5457564/. Accessed 9 Dec 2019

Spiritual Care and Dignity in Old Age

4

Linda Rykkje and Wilfred McSherry

Contents

4.1 Learning Objectives

This chapter will:

- Provide an overview of what is meant by the concepts of spirituality, spiritual/existential care and dignity

L. Rykkje (✉)
Faculty of Health Studies, VID Specialized University, Bergen, Norway
e-mail: Linda.Rykkje@vid.no

W. McSherry
Department of Nursing, School of Health and Social Care, Staffordshire University, Stoke-On-Trent, UK

University Hospitals of North Midlands NHS Trust, Stoke-on-Trent/Stafford, England, UK

Professor VID Specialized University College Bergen/Oslo, Oslo, Norway
e-mail: w.mcsherry@staffs.ac.uk

© Springer Nature Switzerland AG 2021
W. McSherry et al. (eds.), *Understanding Ageing for Nurses and Therapists*,
Perspectives in Nursing Management and Care for Older Adults,
https://doi.org/10.1007/978-3-030-40075-0_4

- Demonstrate how those working in the care of older people can alleviate spiritual and existential suffering
- Offer insights and strategies for safeguarding the dignity of older people

4.2   Introduction

In this chapter, we introduce different views on how spiritual and existential issues may be relevant for older people. Our perspective is that within a holistic nursing and healthcare tradition, we must take care of the whole person, including the physical, psychological, social and spiritual aspects of life. We also find that safeguarding the older persons' dignity presupposes that we respect the uniqueness of each person, acknowledging that our world or life view may be very different from the people we care for and work alongside. We stress the importance of how dignity and respect are fundamental to a person's life view and if applicable, his/her religious beliefs.

Older people are not a homogeneous cohort but are just as different as persons in any other age groups are. When we care for older people, we must have knowledge about different cultures and both non-religious and religious ways of relating to old age and how this may affect the later stages of life. Therefore, we find it of uttermost importance for health and social care professionals to be sensitive to spiritual, religious and existential needs, and to understand what is important for each person, in order to safeguard the patients' dignity. This awareness is important because such values and beliefs may contribute to the alleviation of spiritual or existential distress and suffering.

Spiritual and existential care will be addressed within a Christian-humanistic framework, with openness towards other world views of life and religions. The overall aim of the chapter is to reinforce how respect for older people wishes and an openness to their hopes and fears for the future may contribute to a richer life. Hence, it is our goal that everyday life may become as peaceful and enjoyable as possible.

4.3   Spirituality, Religion and Existential Aspects of Care

Reflective Exercise
- Before we proceed with this section, we would like you to think about the words spiritual, existential and religion. How might these be relevant to the care of older people?
- A useful exercise that might help is to fold an A4 piece of paper into three columns and label the first column spiritual, the second existential and the third religion. Now just write down any thoughts and ideas that come to mind. Do not think about this too much, just what springs to mind and write your thought under the respective column.

These concepts are very personal and subjective since they are related to extremely sensitive and deeply personal aspects of what it is to be a human being. Such matters (areas of life) are often difficult to articulate and describe in any concrete manner. They are also dealing with areas of life that can be very contentious, living in a world that is becoming progressively secular and materialistic. A world that is almost intolerant to any reference or mention to these concepts because of the misconceptions, fears and prejudice that are associated with them. Perhaps you had difficulty in articulating your ideas; this is not unusual because we do not always consciously think about these concepts on a regular or daily basis. Both Rykkje [1] and McSherry [2] found this when they asked patients in their research about the participants' understanding of spirituality. Furthermore, McSherry found that many patients struggled to provide an understanding, many seeing it purely in religious or supernatural terms, such as ghosts and ghouls. Interestingly, when he asked health and social care professionals the same question, they were able to offer quite in-depth, insightful and elaborate understandings.

4.3.1 Spirituality and Religion

We find there are many attempts in the literature to address the concepts of spirituality and religion. Sørensen et al. [3, p. 93] provide a useful distinction:

> Orientations towards an immaterial, supernatural power are considered as "religion" when it occurs as organized with institutional components of faith traditions [4]. "Spirituality" addresses individuals' relationships with and search for the sacred. The sacred refers to God or higher powers, but also other aspects of life perceived as manifestations of the divine or features having divine-like qualities [5].

This quotation implies that 'religion' is expressed within a community context, while 'spirituality' is more individually focused. This approach reflects that of other writing in healthcare. Koenig et al. [6] make a distinction between religion and spirituality (see Table 4.1).

While this table may be useful in differentiating what might constitute religion and spirituality in a formal, institutional sense, it does very little to describe what may be considered the main essence of these concepts. A useful exercise would be for you to reflect upon two definitions of these concepts as used within healthcare.

The authors are aware that a great deal of debate and evidence has been written on these concepts in other disciplines. However, for the purpose of this chapter,

Table 4.1 Distinguishing religion and spirituality

Religion	Spirituality
Community-focused	Individualistic
Observable, measurable, objective	Less visible and measurable, more subjective
Formal orthodox, organized	Less formal, orthodox, less systematic
Behaviour-orientated, outward practices	Emotionally orientated, inward directed
Authoritarian in terms of behaviour	Not authoritarian, little accountability
Doctrine separating good from evil	Unifying, not doctrine-oriented

Adapted from Koenig et al. [6, p. 18]

we draw only upon the work of Murray and Zentner [7, p. 259] who state that 'religion' is:

> A belief in a supernatural or divine force that has power over the universe and commands worship and obedience; a system of beliefs; a comprehensive code of ethics or philosophy; a set of practices that are followed; a church affiliation; the conscious pursuit of any object the person holds as supreme.

A limitation of this definition in contemporary society is the overemphasis on church affiliation, which implies Christianity. Our societies and healthcare are not so monocultural since there are people from all major religions with diverse world views, beliefs, values and ethnic backgrounds. Murray and Zentner [7, p. 259] define spirituality as:

> A quality that goes beyond religious affiliation, that strives for inspirations, reverence, awe, meaning and purpose, even in those who do not believe in any good. The spiritual dimension tries to be in harmony with the universe, and strives for answers about the infinite, and comes into focus when the person faces emotional stress, physical illness or death.

Your reflections may have revealed that there are some shared elements, for example, both appear to focus on the supernatural, the sacred and include beliefs, values and relationships that can have a profound impact on people's everyday lives and existence.

A more recent definition of spirituality being used in healthcare is the one developed by Puchalski et al. [8, p. 646]. This definition was the outcome of an international consensus conference on spirituality. They state spirituality is:

> A dynamic and intrinsic aspect of humanity through which persons seek ultimate meaning, purpose, and transcendence, and experience relationship to self, family, others, community, society, nature, and the significant or sacred. Spirituality is expressed through beliefs, values, traditions, and practices.

Analysis of the definitions of spirituality presented in this chapter reveals that there are common and recurrent attributes present within such definitions. These are often listed as meaning, purpose and fulfilment, transcendence, connection and relations.

4.3.2 Existential

You will notice that so far that we have not attempted to address or define what is meant by the term existential, this omission has been deliberate. What could be termed the primary attributes of spirituality and religion are issues of transcendence, relationships, meaning and purpose, connections and how we communicate with each other. Thus, spirituality and religion are central to and either explicitly or implicitly features the term meaning and purpose. Here, we could also add in the word fulfilment. We find that the existential dimension is influenced by spirituality and religion. DeMarinis [9, pp. 44–45] writing from a religion and psychology perspective suggests:

> The existential dimension is focused on the individual's understanding of existentiality and the way meaning is created. This dimension includes the worldview conception, life approach, decision-making structure, way of relating, and way of understanding. It also includes the activities of expressions of symbolic significance, such as rituals and other ways of making meaning.

As you might notice, this definition of the 'existential' also includes several of the components outlined in religion and spirituality. One observation from all three definitions presented in this section is that they appear to place an emphasis on intellect, rationality and introspection. This may be problematic when we apply these concepts within the care of the older person. Since some older people will not have this capacity, having lost this ability through neuro-degenerative conditions and cognitive impairment in dementia.

4.4   Alleviate Suffering

Reflective Exercise
Before we proceed with this section, we would like you to reflect upon the following questions:

- How do you understand the word suffering?
- Have you encountered suffering in your care of older people?
- It can be useful to think back to a specific patient situation that you remember well because it made an impact upon you. Reflect upon the situation; what happened and could you have done something differently?

The nature of spirituality is linked to the phenomena of suffering and what can be understood as spiritual awakening or desire. This desire can arise both in the face of suffering and in the face of significant life events, such as childbirth, divorce and death [10]. When human beings face illness and adversity in life, spirituality can have a greater significance.

We understand that human suffering is a natural or unavoidable part of life [11]. Eriksson [12] describes three forms of suffering, which is suffering through illness, suffering of life and suffering related to healthcare. We as health and social care workers may cause suffering more than being of help, if we violate patients, abuse our power or fail to deliver care. Suffering related to healthcare could be both caused by the individual caregiver or by the result of organizational or cultural matters [11].

Suffering is commonly linked to experiences of encountering something painful and difficult in life and is, therefore, often associated with illness or adverse life events. According to Eriksson [13, p. 73], suffering is not a feeling or pain in itself, it is more fundamental—'a state of being' [13]. Eriksson points out that the spiritual dimension takes on a deeper meaning in the experience of suffering and that a transition to and emphasis on spirituality is often the most profound response to suffering. Through suffering, spiritual desires may arise, and this leads to an increased awareness in man of his own spirituality. Suffering has no meaning in itself, however, it is possible to find that experiencing suffering can have a purpose [14]. The human being's ability to suffer is a condition for growth, and through suffering one comes in contact with the basic conditions of life.

Our view is that care is not about removing all suffering, but that the care is about the patient experiencing a health condition that is compatible with tolerable suffering. If suffering is understood as a meaningful experience, caregivers may have the opportunity to help the patient gain better insight into their own spiritual needs [13]. The spiritual becomes visible when experiences of suffering are shared with others, and difficult situations can be transformed into a process that results in improved health, well-being and experience of wholeness. Thus, this underscores the need for nurses and social workers to include the spiritual dimension of human beings in their care. Jackson et al. [15] find that healthcare professionals still lack confidence in providing spiritual care and suggest an organizational approach in order to meet older people's need for spiritual care and support.

The goal of spiritual care for older people is to support and promote their health and quality of life, as well as to prevent and alleviate spiritual unrest or suffering. For nursing home residents, spirituality can be considered as a framework for their life experiences, where the spiritual dimension can foster an experience of peacefulness. You might think that alleviation of suffering is rather difficult. However, what you need to reflect upon is how to provide compassionate care and to let yourself be touched in some way by the patient because such care can alleviate suffering [16].

4.5 Dignity and Respect

Reflective Exercise
Before proceeding with this section, we would like you to reflect upon the following questions:

- What is your understanding of the word dignity?
- Why may this concept be important when caring for older people (any person)?

Over the past decade, a great deal of attention has been focused on the concept of dignity in care and how this can contribute to the patients' experience and overall quality of care. Matiti and Baillie [17] explored the concept of dignity within different caring environment and contexts. Tranvåg et al. [18] use a novel, innovative approach to the exploration of dignity by using stories to demonstrate how dignity can be preserved with diverse healthcare setting.

Interestingly, since 2006 in England, there has been a national dignity campaign. This campaign was initially launched by the Department of Health but has been continued by the National Dignity Council and not for profit organization and registered charity. The catalyst for the launch of the campaign and its continuation are some significant failing in care that have been highlighted in both the health and social care sectors in the United Kingdom. The National Dignity Council [19] states:

> The campaign's core values are about having dignity in our hearts, minds and actions, changing the culture of care services and placing a greater emphasis on improving the quality of care and the experience of citizens using services including NHS hospitals, community services, care homes and home support services.

In Norway, the Ministry of Health and Care Services [20] has focused upon dignity in old age, providing a Dignity Guarantee stating that the municipal nursing and care services shall facilitate the care of the elderly, which guarantees the individual recipient a dignified and as meaningful life as possible in accordance with their individual needs.

4.5.1 Dignity in Old Age

Fenton and Mitchell [21, p. 21] provide the following definition of dignity in the context of caring for older people:

> Dignity is a state of physical, emotional and spiritual comfort, with each individual valued for his or her uniqueness and his or her individuality celebrated. Dignity is promoted when individuals are enabled to do the best within their capabilities, exercise control, make choices and feel involved in the decision-making that underpins their care.

This definition reinforces a holistic approach to the delivery of dignified care. There is equal emphasis on all dimensions so the person and the spiritual/existential is not neglected or omitted affirming the importance of this in the provision of person-centred care. It is clear from the above definition that dignity is preserved when older people feel in control are able to make choices, and they are involved in any decision-making processes concerning their care and indeed their lives.

A great deal of attention has been given to the concept of dignity in care, with several models and theories being advocated. Nordenfelt and Edgar [22], as part of a European study exploring older people's perceptions of dignity, developed the four notions of dignity model (see Table 4.2). Table 4.2 was developed summarizing the four notions model as part of the Health and Social Care Advisory Service 'Dignity through action resource guide'. This table provides a useful summary of each of the four notions.

Table 4.2 Four notions of dignity

Dignity of the **human being**	• Conventions and laws
	• Right to life
	• No abuse
	• Justice
	• Privacy
	• No discrimination
	• Freedoms/respect
	   Conscience
	   Religion
	   Expression
	   Association

Dignity of **personal identity**	• Personal identity • Self-respect • Self-esteem • Resilience • Personal relationships
Dignity of **merit**	• Achievements • Rank and seniority • Place in society • Honours awarded • Employment • Knowledge & skills • Experience • Qualifications • Financial worth • Success in life • Independence
Dignity of **moral status**	• People's moral principles • Religious faith • Community membership • Leadership • Recognized roles

Adapted from the Health and Social Care Advisory Service (2010) 'Dignity through action resource guide'.

Reflective Exercise
Spend a few moments reading through the items listed under each of the four notions of dignity.

- What do these tell you about the concept of dignity?
- How might this impact on how we care for older people?

The four notions of dignity model demonstrate and reinforce that every single person should be treated with dignity and respect. Whether this be the person receiving care, their loved ones or family members and indeed the staff who are providing care. Dignity encompasses all of the holistic dimensions of a person, and in many countries of the world, it is protected under Human Rights legislation. Dignity touches at the heart of what it is to be a person and how this is so integral to our sense of identity, self-worth. Dignity involves our personal beliefs, values and relationships since these shape and inform our moral principles and guide our conduct and behaviours.

It should be noted that others have commented on Nordenfelt's model of dignity. Wainwright and Gallagher [23] point to that all human life in all its forms is worthy of respect. They suggest that we simply recognize others as being of worth and that a system of classification that sets up inclusion and exclusion criteria may be a mistake.

In the caring science tradition, dignity is related to respect and autonomy in care [11]. Furthermore, Eriksson [14] perceives all humans as equal and inviolable, and caring must concern the whole person and the confirmation of each person's incalculable worth. If the dignity of the person is violated, the person may experience suffering. Caring for the whole human being means that we must accept the patient's spiritual experiences and alleviate spiritual suffering. As such, there is an interconnection between caring for the spirit and caring for the whole human being, thus aiming to safeguard the patients' dignity. Dignity in care requires that we see the other person the way he or she is, perhaps in the middle of suffering, being accepting and not questioning the person, and also to be responsible for the other person's well-being. Regarding dignity, these are the words of Eriksson [14, p. 73]: 'Every time we meet another person we can, by our attitude, either oppress or confirm the other person, reject or raise him/her to another level of self-respect'.

We assume that aspects of the spiritual dimension; that means what the patients themselves think is important might form a foundation for fostering dignity in old age. Based on interviews of older people, Rykkjc [1] suggests that an important part of spiritual care is to receive love from family and friends through visits and expressions of concern, and that these relationships can be a great source for meaning in older people's lives. Rykkje concludes in her study that the essence of dignity in old age is being confirmed by experiencing being loved, not forgotten, and feeling alive through spiritual care. Nurses should promote the older persons' own resources and the maintenance of their close relationships, and especially support their need to be needed (reciprocity). This we think will support the older persons' personal dignity.

Practice Example
Having explored the meaning of dignity and discussed how spirituality and dignity are interconnected, we would now like to explore the application of these concepts within practice.

Please read the following case taken from The Parliamentary and Health Service Ombudsman [24] report titled Care and Compassion? Report of the Health Service Ombudsman on ten investigations into NHS care of older people:

'Mr D was diagnosed with advanced stomach cancer. His discharge, originally planned for Tuesday 30 August, was brought forward to 27 August, the

Saturday of a bank holiday weekend. On the day of discharge, which his daughter described as a 'shambles', the family arrived to find Mr D in a distressed condition behind drawn curtains in a chair. He had been waiting for several hours to go home. He was in pain, desperate to go to the toilet and unable to ask for help because he was so dehydrated, he could not speak properly or swallow. His daughter told us that 'his tongue was like a piece of dried leather'. The emergency button had been placed beyond his reach. His drip had been removed and the bag of fluid had fallen and had leaked all over the floor making his feet wet. When the family asked for help to put Mr D on the commode he had 'squealed like a piglet' with pain. An ambulance booked to take him home in the morning had not arrived and at 2.30 pm the family decided to take him home in their car. This was achieved with great difficulty and discomfort for Mr D'.

This extract from the case report highlights the fundamental role healthcare professionals play in preserving the dignity of those in their care. It emphasizes that dignity can be violated in so many ways in terms of not communicating effectively with patients and their families, not providing adequate pain management and ensuring arrangements for discharge are made well in advance and actioned responsibly. Jacobson [25] provides a very useful taxonomy of dignity highlighting those attitudes, values and behaviours that can preserve dignity and those that can lead to dignity violation.

4.6 Summary of Main Points

In this chapter, we have provided different views upon spiritual, religious and existential care. We have also pointed to the alleviation of suffering, based on the caring science tradition. Furthermore, we explored the interconnectedness between human dignity and spirituality. Safeguarding the human worth and dignity is of great importance in older people care, and we have suggested some promising strategies. However, we have not looked into specific caring needs of people with dementia. Although there is a small but increasing research-base focusing on both dignity and specific spiritual needs for people who cannot so easily express their own needs, we suggest further research in this area.

4.7 Suggested Reading and Resources

National Dignity Council (2020) Dignity in care campaign Available https://www. dignityincare.org.uk/About/ [Accessed 20-1-2020]

Tranvåg, O., Synnes, O., & McSherry, W. (Eds.) (2016). *Stories of Dignity within Healthcare: Research, narratives and theories.* Keswick: M&K Publishing.

Puchalski, C, M., Vitillo, R., Hull, S, K., Reller, N. (2014) Improving the Spiritual Dimension of Whole Person Care: Reaching National and International Consensus, Journal of Palliative Medicine, 17(6): 642–656.

Jackson, D., Doyle, C., Capon, H., & Pringle, E. (2016). Spirituality, spiritual need, and spiritual care in aged care: What the literature says. *Journal of Religion, Spirituality & Aging*, 28(4), 281–295.

References

1. Rykkje L (2019) Views on spirituality in old age: what does love have to do with it? Religions 10(1):5
2. McSherry W (2007) The meaning of spirituality and spiritual care within nursing and health care practice. Quay Books, Wiltshire
3. Sørensen T, Lien L, Landheim A, Danbolt LJ (2015) Meaning-making, religiousness and spirituality in religiously founded substance misuse services—a qualitative study of staff and patients' experiences. Religions 6:92–106. https://doi.org/10.3390/rel6010092
4. Aldwin CM, Park CL, Jeong YJ, Nath R (2014) Differing pathways between religiousness, spirituality, and health: a self-regulation perspective. Psychol Relig Spiritual 6(1):9
5. Pargament KI, Mahoney A, Exline JJ, Jones JW, Shafranske EP (2013) Envisioning an integrative paradigm for the psychology of religion and spirituality. In: Pargament KI (ed) APA Handbook of psychology, religion, and spirituality. American Psychology Association, Washington, DC, pp 3–19
6. Koenig HG, McCullough ME, Larson DB (2001) Handbook of religion and health. Oxford University Press, Oxford
7. Murray RB, Zentner JB (1989) Nursing concepts for health promotion. Prentice Hall, London
8. Puchalski CM, Vitillo R, Hull SK, Reller N (2014) Improving the spiritual dimension of whole person care: reaching national and international consensus. J Palliat Med 17(6):642–656
9. DeMarinis V (2008) The impact of Postmodernization on existential health in Sweden: psychology of religion's function in existential public health analysis. Arch Psychol Relig 30:57–74
10. Rykkje L, Eriksson K, Råholm M-B (2011) A qualitative metasynthesis of spirituality from a caring science perspective. Int J Hum Caring 15(4):40–53
11. Arman M, Ranheim A, Rydenlund K, Rytterström P, Rehnsfeldt A (2015) The Nordic tradition of caring science: the works of three theorists. Nurs Sci Q 28(4):288–296
12. Eriksson K (2006) The suffering human being. Nordic Studies Press, Chicago
13. Råholm M.-B, Lindholm L, Eriksson K. (2002) Grasping the essence of the spiritual dimension reflected through the horizon of suffering: An interpretative research synthesis. The Australian Journal of Holistic Nursing. 9(1):4–13.
14. Eriksson K (1997) Caring, spirituality and suffering. In: Roach IMS (ed) Caring from the heart: The convergence of caring and spirituality. Paulist Press, New York, pp 68–83
15. Jackson D, Doyle C, Capon H, Pringle E (2016) Spirituality, spiritual need, and spiritual care in aged care: what the literature says. J Relig Spiritual Aging 28(4):281–295
16. Lindholm L, Eriksson K (1993) To understand and alleviate suffering in a caring culture. J Adv Nurs 18(9):1354–1361. https://doi.org/10.1046/j.1365-2648.1993.18091354.x
17. Matiti MR, Baillie L (eds) (2011) Dignity in healthcare: a practical approach for nurses and midwives. Radcliffe Publishing, London
18. Tranvåg O, Synnes O, McSherry W (eds) (2016) Stories of dignity within healthcare: research, narratives and theories. M&K Publishing, Keswick
19. National Dignity Council (2020) Dignity in care campaign. https://www.dignityincare.org.uk/About/. Accessed 20 Jan 2020

20. Ministry of Health and Care Services (2010) Ordinance (No. 1426 of 2010) on a dignified care for the elderly (dignity guarantee). https://lovdata.no/dokument/SF/forskrift/2010-11-12-1426. Accessed 24 Feb 2020
21. Fenton E, Mitchell T (2002) Growing old with dignity: a concept analysis. Nurs Older People 14(4):19
22. Nordenfelt L, Edgar A (2005) The four notions of dignity. Qual Ageing Older Adults 6(1):17–21. https://doi.org/10.1108/14717794200500004
23. Wainwright P, Gallagher A (2008) On different types of dignity in nursing care: a critique of Nordenfelt. Nurs Philos 9(1):46–54
24. The Parliamentary and Health Service Ombudsman (2011) Care and Compassion? Available from https://www.ombudsman.org.uk/sites/default/files/2016-10/Care%20and%20Compassion.pdf [Accessed 22/03/2021]
25. Jacobson N (2009) A taxonomy of dignity: a grounded theory study. BMC Int Health Hum Rights 9(1):3. https://doi.org/10.1186/1472-698X-9-3

The Psychology of Ageing

5

Linn-Heidi Lunde

Contents

5.1 Learning Objectives

This chapter will provide you with knowledge about how to:

- Understand the normal age-related changes associated with cognition
- Examine the concept of personality highlighting how this may change because of normal ageing
- Explore issues related to coping and control, and how these may be effected by normal ageing processes

L.-H. Lunde (✉)
Department of Addiction Medicine, Haukeland University Hospital, Bergen, Norway
e-mail: linn-heidi.lunde@uib.no

© Springer Nature Switzerland AG 2021
W. McSherry et al. (eds.), *Understanding Ageing for Nurses and Therapists*,
Perspectives in Nursing Management and Care for Older Adults,
https://doi.org/10.1007/978-3-030-40075-0_5

5.2   Introduction

Health and social care professionals like nurses, social workers and care assistant
working with older people need up-to-date information and empirical knowledge
about normal ageing processes to provide best practice treatment and care to their
older patients. In order to combat common myths and negative stereotypes about
ageing such as exaggerated attitudes about decline and frailty, it is important to
acquire a nuanced perspective that shows the complexity of ageing, and not the
least, the diversity of ageing. We should also keep in mind that new cohorts of older
people are healthier than previous cohorts and that increased longevity does not
necessarily means increased disability [1].

5.2.1   A Lifespan Perspective on Ageing

Ageing is a lifelong and gradual process that starts at birth and lasts all life [2]. First
and foremost, ageing means change, and the changes occur biologically, psychologically, socially and culturally, and these processes affect each other mutually.
Decline and growth take place at the same time throughout the life cycle. One example is how the brain weakens and deteriorates when it is not sufficiently stimulated,
while new experience such as physical and mental exercise helps to improve brain
function in young as well as in old age [3].

Ageing and growing older have to be considered as part of a long life, where past
events, living conditions and choices one has taken will shape old age [2]. An
important characteristic of older people is the heterogeneity and the large individual
diversity in how older people appear and function. People age in different ways and
at a different pace, and various life burdens and living conditions influence the ageing process. The birth cohort one belongs to and the historical time in which one
grows up will characterize who each of us become as elderly. Unfortunately, most
people tend to regard older people as a homogeneous group that are similar to one
another and have the same needs. However, the second half of life is characterized
by a great diversity and large individual differences in terms of health, functioning,
interests, habits and preferences.

5.2.2   The Psychology of Ageing: What Is It?

Normal psychological ageing involves changes in mental processes such as cognition, personality and emotional functioning and behaviour throughout the life cycle
[1]. Psychological ageing is closely related to biological ageing, but also to the
changes that occur in the environment's expectations of the individual as a result of
increased chronological age. Thus, psychological ageing is also about adapting to
biological ageing and social expectations [1].

This chapter will review and discuss normal age-related changes in cognition,
personality, emotions, coping and control and how such changes may affect the

function of everyday life. A case vignette has been designed to illustrate such changes (see Box 5.1 below). The reader should bear in mind that the psychological changes are intertwined with biological and physical changes, which are covered in Chap. 2 (Physiology and ageing).

Box 5.1

It is Ann's birthday and she is 78 years old. Ann has invited her closest family and some friends to the celebration. The party takes place in her son's house, and the practical details are being taken care of by a catering company. Ann thinks it's a relief not to have to make dinner for so many guests. She has less energy for such tasks now. What has happened over the years that have passed? Ann feels pretty much like the one she's always been. At least on the inside. She has noticed some improvements though. She gets less annoyed and doesn't take things as seriously as she did when she was younger. These are signs of maturation, Ann thinks. Moreover, she feels much more confident about herself and who she is, compared to when she was younger.

Ann looks at herself in the mirror. She thinks she looks wiser and calmer than she did earlier in her life. The nice dress she wears fits her in a neatly way. She has always been slim thanks to regular physical activity and she is still in quite good shape. It is nice to feel that the body works well, it is good for her self-esteem. Ann replaces a hearing aid in her right ear. It's so tiny this new appliance and quite difficult to handle. However, it makes conversation easier. Ann's hearing has gradually deteriorated, and this is something that Ann really expected because her father had severely impaired hearing when he was an old man. Ann is happy that she has no particular memory problems yet. She notices that she needs more time to recall names, but she eventually remembers. Ann believes that reading books, solving crosswords and Sudoku are activities that will help to prevent memory problems. She thinks she is doing well in many ways, but she misses her husband George who passed away 5 years ago.

At the end of the chapter, a short review of the most common mental health problems in older adults as well as a description of intellectual disability and old age will be provided.

Reflective Questions
1. In the vignette, the maturation of the emotional life in old age is highlighted. Why is this aspect important and what are the consequences of emotional maturity in old age?
2. At the age of 78, Ann shows signs of both decline and growth. Reflect upon how health and social care professionals can motivate and support older persons to prevent premature functional decline.

3. In the story about Ann, she seems to deal with her challenges independently and has a good life. What do you understand as Ann's main challenges in old age? As a professional, you might have met others with
similar challenges and who struggle in their everyday life. Reflect upon
how older people cope with and solve their challenges differently, and if
and how professionals or others can be of assistance.

5.3 Changes in Cognition

Cognition includes phenomena such as sensory perception, attention, memory,
thinking, problem-solving and intelligence [4]. Changes in brain structure and
changes in cognitive abilities and function occur at the same time throughout life.
Many of the cognitive changes occur slowly and gradually. One example is the reaction capability or the time it takes to respond to stimuli (speed of processing). The
reaction time or capability is increasing from the age of 20, which means that it will
gradually take longer to perceive, process and respond to information. In older
adults, impaired responsiveness can affect skills such as operating machines in the
workplace and driving motor vehicles. However, in most healthy older people, such
changes will have minor impact on daily life [4]. There are also large individual
variations in the course of ageing and functional decline, as mentioned above.

5.3.1 Sensory Perception and Attention

The way the individual perceives and interprets sensory information depends on
how the sensory apparatus (sight, hearing, smell, taste and touch) work, but also the
brain's ability to register and organize the sensory information. With increasing age,
changes and decline take place in the sensory apparatus like reduced vision and
hearing, and stronger stimulation is needed to perceive and interpret sensory information [5]. Everyday examples are that some people need to spice up their food
more than before or have to compensate for sensory loss by using a hearing aid like
Ann in the case presented in the vignette. Understanding and interpreting sensory
information also depends on being alert and able to hold on to an activity without
being distracted or disturbed. The ability to pay attention to multiple tasks at the
same time (so-called divided attention) as required, for example, in complex actions
such as driving, is declining as you grow older. However, the consequences of such
age-related changes might be minimized by adapting and accommodating to such
declines, for example, to avoid driving at night.

5.3.2 Memory

Memory is a very complex function, and in cognitive psychology various memory
systems or subgroups of memory are described [4]. The distinction is made, among
other things, between working memory or short-term memory and long-term

memory and between implicit and explicit memory. Working memory and short-term memory are often used synonymously. Working memory has a limited capacity of seconds, exactly the time needed to remember a telephone number. This form of memory is gradually declining, from a young adult age. With increasing age, it takes longer to understand and process information, and one must concentrate to a greater extent than before to remember or recall information.

There are various forms of long-term memory. Explicit memory (also called declarative memory) is information that the individual has conscious access to, and which demands attention and concentration. Semantic memory is about recalling factual knowledge such as European capitals. This form of memory remains stable or improves throughout life. Episodic memory is to remember special events and experiences, such as 9/11 (i.e. the 11th September 2001 when the Twin Towers in New York were hit by terrorists). This form of long-term memory is declining by age so that older adults have greater difficulty remembering time and place for certain events/episodes than younger adults. Implicit memory, also called procedural memory, involves unconscious access to information. This form of memory involves skills and routine activities that have been automatized, such as cycling, swimming, reading and dancing. Such skills do not require remembering the context in which the skills were acquired and are, therefore, only slightly affected by ageing [4].

With increasing age, it becomes more difficult to remember spontaneously, for example, to recall names, just like Ann experiences in the vignette. When it comes to recognizing, on the other hand, that is, remembering by means of cues in the surroundings, there are no differences between older and younger adults [4]. For example, to remember episodes and stories from your schooldays when you look at an old photo of your classmates. It is also important to be aware that factors other than age may also affect memory, such as health problems and stress, whether you are tired, hungry or use medications that affect memory like, for example, benzodiazepines [4]. In addition, memories that are stored when you are happy, scared or angry will be remembered better than more neutral events. Also, an individual's expectations that memory declines with age could affect the ability to recall. The common stereotype held by many people that ageing involves cognitive decline in memory and learning can become a self-fulfilling prophecy [6]. You may use less effort or energy to remember if you believe memory declines with age or that it is difficult or impossible to acquire new skills as you grow older. The consequences may be impaired cognitive function or at worst, serious cognitive decline [6]. In a recently published study, Levy and her co-workers found that negative stereotypes about ageing have an impact on brain structures and may contribute to pathological changes as in Alzheimer's disease [7]. Conversely, a more optimistic approach like Ann's, with the belief that it is possible to influence cognitive functioning by stimulation and exercise, can slow down the ageing process [6], which will be discussed in Sect. 5.3.5 below.

5.3.3   Learning and Intelligence

Intelligence is closely related to memory and learning, but also includes thinking and problem-solving. Put simply, intelligence in daily life is about the ability to learn and the ability to use what one has learned. With ageing, there is a certain decline in intelligence as measured by intelligence tests. There is a distinction between what is called fluid intelligence and crystallized or fixed intelligence. Fluid intelligence is about the ability to quickly perceive and process information and to see new connections. This kind of intelligence reaches a peak in young adulthood. Crystallized intelligence, on the other hand, is the ability to use knowledge that is accumulated through experience and maturity. This form of intelligence shows a high degree of stability throughout life [4].

5.3.4 Brain Plasticity and Cognitive Reserve

Previously, it was believed that no new nerve cells and nerve cell connections were formed in the ageing brain. In recent decades, neuroscience and the development of advanced brain imaging techniques have given us new knowledge and insights about the brain and its function and capacity [8]. This knowledge has shown us that the brain is plastic, which means that it has a great potential for change, not least through exercise and new experience [8]. This occurs in both young and old brains. Moreover, during the life course, the individual accumulates a cognitive reserve that works protective against the development of impairment and disease [3]. An example of whether a person has high or low cognitive reserve is education level, and longer education can thus protect against the development of cognitive decline and diseases like dementia [3]. Education generally increases skills and the ability to take control of one's life. Highly educated people seek out to a greater extent information that is important in preventing health problems, such as making the right lifestyle choices. Furthermore, highly educated people usually have good finances and, therefore, can afford to pay for what is health promoting.

5.3.5 Cognitive Training and Stimulation

Like all functions in older years, there is great diversity and great individual variations in cognitive capacity and functioning. Cognitive functions are largely influenced by lifestyle factors such as intellectual and social stimulation, but also by physical activity [8]. In addition, it is important to have a balanced diet, moderate intake of alcohol and to avoid smoking and medications that affect cognitive function (e.g. regular use of benzodiazepines and opioids). Such lifestyle choices are crucial in reducing the consequences of normal age-related changes, but also in preventing pathological conditions in the brain and possibly some forms of dementia. Research has shown that systematic exercise and training of cognitive functions, such as memory, has a good effect in healthy older adults [3]. This can be done in various ways, such as learning memory techniques, but just as important are everyday activities such as physical activity, socializing, reading, solving crosswords or doing crafts. Health and social care workers should encourage their older patients to engage themselves in such activities to prevent premature cognitive decline.

5.4   Personality Throughout the Lifespan

Ageing and growing older is often associated with changes in personality, most often in a stereotype and negative way. Like becoming a grumpy and rigid old man or woman unwilling to change views and habits. Research on personality and personality development throughout life is characterized by great diversity, where different models and theories have used different definitions and operationalizations of the concept of personality. The following section will review two of these theories.

5.4.1   Erikson's Theory of Personality Development

One of the most well-known theories of personality is the Swiss psychoanalyst Erik Erikson's theory of human development throughout life [9]. The theory argues that the individual faces different challenges at different life stages, which must be addressed. The individual's way of dealing or coping with the challenges may have consequences for the next stage of development or life phase. Erikson believed that the greatest challenge in old age is accepting the course of life and the choices one has made throughout life and preparing for life to end. If the individual accepts his/her life for good and for bad, this will contribute to a wider perspective on life and to wisdom, which Erikson referred to as ego integrity. Conversely, failing to reconcile or regret the choices one has made can lead to despair and an experience of having failed in life. Which in turn can lead to impaired health and quality of life in older years. While Erikson's model gives us a more general understanding of personality throughout life, other models have been most concerned with personality as having different traits or characteristics.

5.4.2   Five-Factor Model of Personality

The personality theory that may have the most impact today is the so-called Five-Factor model, also called "The Big Five" [10]. The Five-Factor model focuses on personality as consisting of different traits that can be measured and described using personality tests [10]. The personality traits cannot predict what the individual will do in individual situations but are primarily indicators of what behaviour or action is likely/unlikely [11]. The Five-factor model is based on five basic personality dimensions (in the next section, these will be related to Ann in the vignette):

1. Neuroticism: covering various negative emotions such as being moody and worrying
2. Extroversion: which involves being social, outgoing and confident
3. Openness to Experience: which means that one is open to new experiences, is curious and has an active imagination
4. Agreeableness: a trait associated with being warm, generous and helpful
5. Conscientiousness: that one is concerned with being organized and having self-discipline

5.4.3   Stability and Change in Personality and Emotions

According to the Five-factor model, personality and personality traits remain consistently stable throughout life [10]. Just like Ann in the case vignette who feels pretty much like the person she has always been. There are still some age-related changes, but these are considered to be relatively modest. Growing older seems to lead to emotional stability with less neuroticism, which results in fewer negative emotions, but also less extroversion, less openness to new experiences and more warmth and conscientiousness. Such stability and maturation of the emotional life in old age have been documented in several studies [12, 13], and it has been argued that older people are, therefore, more resilient than younger ones [14]. They are less overwhelmed by external stress, and such increase in emotional adjustment and regulation contributes in turn to a greater degree of emotional well-being [14]. Some explanations given are that a long life gives us greater knowledge about ourselves and strengthens our ability to deal with stressful situations as we age. Because the future perspective is limited by increasing age, older people will become more involved in thoughts and behaviours that promote emotional well-being. For many, this can serve as protection against the development of mental disorders in old age [15].

People are different from each other regarding the stability of their personality across the lifespan. In some people, larger changes occur than in others [11]. Various life events and life experiences such as health problems, loss of loved ones, divorce or becoming unemployed can effect personality and cause changes such as less extroversion and more neuroticism or emotional instability [11]. However, such changes are largely transient and reversible. Lasting changes in personality are primarily related to severe mental disorders or organic brain disorders such as dementia [11]. But, lasting personality changes can also occur because of self-development through, for example, psychotherapy. Using psychological methods and tools may help a person to change negative thought patterns and achieve greater emotional stability and less neuroticism [16].

5.4.4   Personality and Health

Negative stereotypes about ageing can, as mentioned above, affect cognitive function, but also health and mortality. A variety of studies on personality and mortality in old age have, in line with Levy's research [6, 7], documented that certain personality traits have negative effects on health and quality of life in older years, especially neuroticism and being low on extroversion and conscientiousness [16, 17]. Those who have negative expectations associated with ageing, as well as a tendency for introversion and carelessness, will be at greater risk of health problems and disability in old age [16]. This knowledge is important, not least regarding the prevention of age-related diseases and functional decline. Health and social care workers should be aware of negative self-stereotypes and beliefs in older patients and provide education about the negative effects of such stereotypes and teach them alternative coping strategies. We will now turn to how older people adapt to and cope with the changes taking place in old age.

5.5   Coping and Sense of Control

A common belief is that with age one loses control over several aspects of life. Such a view is largely rooted in stereotypes and negative attitudes towards ageing, which may have negative consequences for health and behaviour, as outlined above. People are different when it comes to experiencing control over a situation. Some believe that there are things that can be done to influence the ageing process like Ann in the case vignette, while others feel that they have less influence, or that the opportunities for control are limited. In general, studies show that perceived control or sense of control declines with age [18, 19]. This is understandable since many of the changes that occur during ageing are not possible to control like loss of a loved one or health-related issues in old age.

However, there are large individual differences in sense of control within an age group and within the same person over time. On average, older adults seem to maintain a general sense of control perhaps in part because they adjust their goals and standards to the situation they are in.

5.5.1   Coping and Coping Strategies

Coping is defined as the way a person acts in a stressful or challenging situation [20]. In old age, coping is largely about adapting to the changes that occurs physically, mentally and socially. According to Lazarus and Folkman [20], there are two main ways to deal with stress and challenges: so-called problem-focused and emotion-focused coping. Problem-focused coping involves changing what causes problems, while emotion-focused coping means changing the perception of what is causing problems. Older people seem to use more emotion-focused coping by lowering their expectations, and they rely on daily routines to reduce the likelihood of problems and stress and to compensate for loss and decline. Ann, for example, compensates for hearing loss by using hearing aid so that she can participate in conversations with several people present.

5.5.2   Sense of Control

Studies show that a strong sense of control is associated with better cognitive functioning, good health and emotional well-being [19, 21]. A strong sense of control can act as a protection in the face of impaired health and other losses in older years. People who initially have a low sense of control, on the other hand, are more vulnerable to the changes that old age can entail. It can lead to less involvement in more appropriate coping strategies such as physical activity and mental training. Women seem to have a lower sense of control than men, but such gender differences are less pronounced in highly educated [19]. Those with low education and low income report less sense of control over their lives than those with good finances and education [18]. Since new generations of older people have a higher level of education compared to previous generations, we can assume that this will have an impact on coping and sense of control. Still, there can be a difficult balance between experiencing control and taking control of various aspects (e.g. making lifestyle changes) on the one hand, and on the other hand also having to recognize that some aspects of ageing cannot be controlled [22]. One such aspect is the increased vulnerability to loss and illness as one gets older. The next section will briefly review the most common mental health problems/disorders in older years and outline some possible interventions and strategies.

5.6   Mental Health Problems in Old Age

Although many older people nowadays are in better health than previous generations, there is nevertheless an increased vulnerability to being affected by illness with increasing age. This applies both to physical and mental illness. In addition to neurocognitive disorders like Alzheimer's disease and other dementias, symptoms of depression and anxiety are the most common mental health problems in older adults [23]. Sleep problems and chronic pain are often accompanying depression and anxiety, and these symptoms mutually exacerbate one another. Furthermore, anxiety and depressive symptoms are often concomitant with severe somatic illness and neurocognitive disorders, and may exacerbate these. The consequences of anxiety and depression in older adults are often devastating and associated with decreased physical, cognitive and social functioning, which in turn leads to impaired quality of life and at worst increased mortality [23].

International studies show that an increasing number of older adults misuse alcohol and medications at a higher rate than previous generations [24, 25]. For many people, alcohol and psychoactive medications like benzodiazepines and sedatives are ways of coping with depressive thoughts and emotions. Due to age-related changes, older adults are more vulnerable to the physiological effects of alcohol and medications. Alcohol misuse and combining alcohol with psychoactive medication can lead to negative health effects, increasing risk of injuries and falls, as well as exacerbating existing mental health problems [24].

5.6.1   Risk Factors

Risk factors for mental health problems and substance misuse in older adults comprise complex interactions among genetic vulnerabilities and age-related neurobiological changes, physical illness and disability, as well as stressful events like loss and bereavement, loneliness and lack of social support [23]. As mentioned above, negative expectations associated with ageing may also contribute to the development of health problems and functional decline in older adults [6].

5.6.2 Preventive Strategies

Health and social care professionals can employ a number of strategies and interventions preventing the development of mental health problems and substance misuse in older people. For example, nurses, social workers and domiciliary care workers can help to encourage and motivate their older patients to make lifestyle changes that will have a positive impact on their mental health and physical well-being, for example, advising about changing their drinking habits and increasing their activity level. First and foremost, negative self-stereotypes like "I am too old to make changes" or "I am too old to exercise" should be challenged. Furthermore, based on common everyday activities, health and social care workers should inform their older patients of the benefits of physical activities and cognitive training and stimulation. See Sect. 5.3.5 above for examples of everyday activities.

5.6.3 Treatment

For older adults being diagnosed with anxiety, depression and/or substance use disorders, there are evidence-based treatments available [23, 24]. Both forms of psychotherapy and psychological interventions like cognitive behavioural therapy and life review therapy have proven effective in older adults. However, studies show that there are still under-detection and under-treatment of mental disorders in the older population [23, 24].

5.6.4 Intellectual Disability and Ageing

As in the general population, life expectancy has increased among people with intellectual disabilities (ID) and many will reach old age. People with ID constitute a heterogeneous population, where Down syndrome is the most common cause of disability [26]. A common feature of people with ID is that ageing starts at a younger age than in the general population. Age-related conditions such as vision and hearing impairments occur in early adulthood, and mental health problems such as anxiety and depression are more frequent in people with ID than in the general population. Furthermore, persons with ID have a higher risk to develop early onset dementia [26]. Some of the health conditions that could have been prevented or treated in persons with ID remain undetected by healthcare services [26]. This is largely due to a lack of knowledge about ageing in people with ID. Health and social care professionals working with people with ID need basic knowledge about ageing and ID. They should be able to support and motivate their patients to take part in activities that may prevent or slow down functional decline, as well as prevent various health conditions related to old age. People with ID need stimulation and training much the same way as the general population. However, they are dependent on being closely followed up by their surroundings to a much larger extent than people in general.

5.7   Summary of Main Points

The objective of this chapter was to provide the reader with insight into normal age-related changes in cognition, personality and coping and control. Furthermore, the heterogeneity and great diversity in old age is emphasized, and that development and decline are parallel processes throughout the lifespan. I have illustrated that negative self-stereotypes about frailty and decay in old age can serve as self-fulfilling prophecies leading to impaired health and functioning. I also offer some strategies for preventing premature decay and illness such as encouraging mental and physical exercise and training and being engaged in regular everyday activities.

5.8   Suggested Reading

Carstensen, L et al. Emotional experience improves with age: evidence based on over 10 years of experience sampling. Psychol Aging. 2011; 26(1): 21–33.

Levy BR. Mind matters. Cognitive and physical effects of aging self-stereotypes. J Gerontol B Psychol Sci Soc Sci. 2003; 58B(4): 203–2011.

Coppus, A.M.W. People with intellectual disability: What do we know about adulthood and life expectancy? Dev Disabil Res Rev. 2013; 18:616.

References

1. Coleman PG, O'Hanlon A (2004) Ageing and development: theories and research. Oxford University Press, New York, p 244
2. Kessler EM, Kruse A, Werner-Dahl H (2014) Clinical geropsychology. A lifespan perspective. In: Pachana NA, Laidlaw K (eds) The Oxford handbook of clinical geropsychology. Oxford University Press, Oxford, pp 3–25
3. de Lange AMG, Sjøli Bråthen AC, Rohani DA, Grydeland H, Fjell AM, Walhovd KB (2017) The effects of memory training on behavioral and microstructural plasticity in young and older adults. Hum Brain Mapp 38(11):5666–5680
4. Zöllig J, Martin M, Schumacher V (2014) Cognitive development in ageing. In: Pachana NA, Laidlaw K (eds) The Oxford handbook of clinical geropsychology. Oxford University Press, Oxford, pp 125–144
5. Margrain TH, Boulton M (2005) Sensory impairment. In: Johnson ML (ed) The Cambridge handbook of age and ageing. Cambridge University Press, Cambridge, pp 121–130
6. Levy BR (2003) Mind matters. Cognitive and physical effects of aging self-stereotypes. J Gerontol B Psychol Sci Soc Sci 58B(4):203–2011

7. Levy BR, Ferucci L, Zonderman AB, Slade MD, Tronocoso J, Resnick SM (2015) A culture-brain link: negative age stereotypes predict Alzheimer's disease biomarkers. Psychol Aging 31(1):82–88
8. Engvig A, Fjell AM, Westlye LT, Moberget T, Sundseth Ø, Larsen VA et al (2010) Effects of memory training on cortical thickness in the elderly. Neuroimage 52(4):1667–1676
9. Erikson EH, Erikson JM, Kivnick HQ (1986) Vital involvement in old age: the experience of old age in our time. Norton, New York, p 352
10. McCrae RR, Costa PT (2003) Personality in adulthood, a five-factor theory perspective, 2nd edn. Guidford Press, New York, p 261
11. Chopik WJ, Kitayama S (2018) Personality change across the life span: insights from a cross-cultural, longitudinal study. J Pers 86:508–521
12. Carstensen L, Pasubathi M, Mayr U, Nesselroade JR (2000) Emotional experience in everyday life across the adult life span. J Pers Soc Psychol 79:644–655
13. Löckenhoff CE, Costa PT, Lane RD (2008) Age differences in description of emotional experience in oneself and others. J Gerontol B Psychol Sci Soc Sci 63:92–99
14. Carstensen L et al (2011) Emotional experience improves with age: evidence based on over 10 years of experience sampling. Psychol Aging 26(1):21–33
15. Blazer D (2010) Protection from late life depression. Int Psychogeriatr 23(2):171–173
16. Mroczek DK, Spiro A, Griffin PW (2006) Personality and aging. In: Birren JE, Schaie KW (eds) Handbook of the psychology of aging. Academic Press, San Diego, pp 363–377
17. Rasmussen HN, Scheier MF, Greenhouse JB (2009) Optimism and physical health: a meta-analytic review. Ann Behav Med 37(3):239–256
18. Lachman ME, Weaver SL (1998) The sense of control as a moderator of social class differences in health and wellbeing. J Pers Soc Psychol 74:763–773
19. Lachman ME, Neupert SD, Agrigoroaei S (2011) The relevance of control beliefs for health and aging. In: Schaie KW, Willis SL (eds) Handbook of the psychology of aging. Academic Press, San Diego, pp 175–190
20. Lazarus RS, Folkman S (1984) Stress, appraisal and coping. Springer, New York, p 456
21. Caplan LJ, Schooler C (2003) The roles of fatalism, self-confidence and intellectual resources in the disablement process in older adults. Psychol Aging 18:551–561
22. Heckhausen J, Wrosch C, Schulz R (2010) A motivational theory of life-span development. Psychol Rev 117(1):32–60
23. Fiske A, Wetherell JL, Gatz M (2009) Depression in older adults. Annu Rev Clin Psychol 5:363–389
24. Barry KL, Blow FC (2016) Drinking across the lifespan: focus on older adults. Alcohol Res 38(1):115–120
25. Caputo F, Vignoli T, Leggio L, Addolorato G, Zoli G, Bernardi M (2012) Alcohol use disorders in the elderly: a brief overview from epidemiology to treatment options. Exp Gerontol 47(6):411–416
26. Coppus AMW (2013) People with intellectual disability: What do we know about adulthood and life expectancy? Dev Disabil Res Rev 18:616

Sexual Intimacy and Ageing

6

Dawne Garrett

Contents

6.1 Learning Objectives

This chapter will enable you to:

- Understand the health and social aspects of sexual ageing
- Examine the barriers and enablers to promoting sexual intimacy
- Explore the clinical interventions that promote healthy sexual ageing

D. Garrett (✉)
Royal College of Nursing, London, UK
e-mail: dawne.garrett@rcn.org.uk

© Springer Nature Switzerland AG 2021
W. McSherry et al. (eds.), *Understanding Ageing for Nurses and Therapists*,
Perspectives in Nursing Management and Care for Older Adults,
https://doi.org/10.1007/978-3-030-40075-0_6

6.2   Introduction

Expressions of sexuality are a normal, natural and positive dimension of healthy ageing; they are an expression of personhood and can be life-affirming. Sexuality is a central characteristic of being human. Maslow [1] identified a hierarchy of human needs, and sex is identified as a "basic" or "physiological" need of a human being. People can remain sexually intimate throughout their lives, but age-related changes are complex and sexual activity changes.

Sexual health in later life confers benefits on general health and quality of life, and sexual intimacy is an enriching part of the lives of many older people with both long-term and new relationships being something that can bring joy and pleasure. As people grow older in sociological terms, they accumulate positive, negative or neutral life transitions; they also age biologically and psychologically, incorporating pathological changes into their life course. Whilst social structures and institutions change, over time, so do populations, technology and social norms, and there is an interactivity between these factors [2]. Older people have never lived so long and many enjoy an excellent quality of life, although it must be acknowledged that living with two or more long-term conditions is common [3]. Retirement extends for a longer period than it has ever done before, and many older people have greater opportunities for time and privacy to enjoy each other's company and to express their feelings for each other [4]. Additionally, older people are now seen as consumers of new and exciting goods and services such as holidays, aesthetic innovations and functional adaptations [5].

However, sexual intimacy remains a topic which many healthcare professionals fail to explore in their clinical practice with older people. All aspects of sexual health form an area which is frequently avoided, with many excuses being put forward as to why it should not be discussed or clinically assessed. These include the idea that it is "too embarrassing for them" or intrusive and unprofessional, or sometimes because we would not know how to respond if the person raised an issue. In this chapter, we will look at the physiological changes which occur in sexual ageing, recognising that the progression and impact are highly individual. Similarly, we will identify the impact of societal norms that influence how older people display their sexuality and address their sexual health. As healthcare professionals, we need to understand our bias and beliefs about sexual intimacy in later life, exploring expectations and possible interventions. There are many barriers and facilitators to healthy sexual ageing, and there are established rights to sexual health for everyone. We need the knowledge and skills to promote sexual health for older people.

6.3   Sexual Intimacy in Older Age

Older people have seen and continue to see huge changes in the nature of sexual expression through their lives. There is increased freedom to be themselves and to consider their sexual activity in myriad ways. In the UKI, there has been a rise in divorce and remarriage, increasing numbers of people living in partnerships both hetero and homosexual and new fluid relationships that include the choice not to cohabit. The availability, nature and effectiveness of contraception, treatment for sexual difficulties and sexually transmitted infections (STIs) have all increased through the lifespan. Older people have experienced expansion in the awareness of sexuality, dating and intergenerational marriage [6]. Many of the earlier social and moral taboos have been removed. However, the stereotypical ideal image of the nuclear family persists, and the heteronormative family ideal, with clear gendered roles, remains even today. Nevertheless, relationships are changing, particularly for older people, and the previous economic imperative of partnerships is giving way to relationships that are more equal and supported. Older people have seen many adjustments in gendered activities, technological and medical innovations, increasing independence of women, changes in the function and role of marriage, increased education and understanding of sexual activities. In short, they have witnessed some of the greatest changes experienced in social history within the UK. Their ability to change, respond and create social mores is hugely significant.

Alongside the cultural and clinical developments, a rights-based approach to sexual intimacy has emerged, championed by the World Health Organisation [7], with clear definition and aspirations. WHO has set out some working definitions to inform the debate about sexual activity in the twenty-first century, which are set out below.

6.3.1 Sex

Sex refers to the biological characteristics that define humans as female or male. While these sets of biological characteristics are not mutually exclusive, as there are individuals who possess both, they tend to differentiate humans as males and females [8].

6.3.2 Sexual Health

According to the current WHO working definition, sexual health is:

> …a state of physical, emotional, mental and social well-being in relation to sexuality; it is not merely the absence of disease, dysfunction or infirmity. Sexual health requires a positive and respectful approach to sexuality and sexual relationships, as well as the possibility of having pleasurable and safe sexual experiences, free of coercion, discrimination and violence. For sexual health to be attained and maintained, the sexual rights of all persons must be respected, protected and fulfilled [9: 3].

6.3.3 Sexual Rights

There is a growing consensus that sexual health cannot be achieved and maintained without respect for, and protection of, certain human rights. The working definition of sexual rights given below is a WHO contribution to the continuing dialogue on human rights related to sexual health. The fulfilment of sexual health is tied to the extent to which human rights are respected, protected and fulfilled. Sexual rights embrace certain human rights that are already recognised in international and regional human rights documents and other consensus documents and in national laws.

Rights critical to the realisation of sexual health include:

- The rights to equality and non-discrimination
- The right to be free from torture or to cruel, inhumane or degrading
- The right to privacy
- The rights to the highest attainable standard of health (including sexual health) and social security
- The right to marry and to find a family and enter into marriage with the free and full consent of the intending spouses, and to equality in and at the dissolution of marriage
- The right to decide the number and spacing of one's children
- The rights to information, as well as education
- The rights to freedom of opinion and expression
- The right to an effective remedy for violations of fundamental rights
- Treatment or punishment

The responsible exercise of human rights requires that all persons respect the rights of others. Older people are often not aware of their healthcare rights, and their entitlement to sexual activities may not be something they have considered before. Therefore, it can be helpful to share these rights with colleagues and individuals to help raise awareness.

6.4   Physiological Changes Relating to Sexual Activity

It is widely recognised that there is individuality in the extent and timing of physical changes in older age. In addition, the more sexually active the person is, the fewer the changes the person is likely to experience in his or her pattern of sexual response [10].

6.4.1   Changes in the Female Body

During the life course, the normal reduction of testosterone, which occurs in all genders, has profound effects. Testosterone supports the libido and is produced by the testes and ovaries; however, for several years after the menopause, the ovaries also supply small amounts of testosterone as well as oestrogen and androstenedione; a decrease in serum testosterone is seen to parallel a decline in libido [6].

The physical changes most frequently commented upon in relation to the female body are the decline in oestrogen production and its implications for urogenital ageing [11]. Urogential ageing is particularly associated with vaginal dryness and atrophy. The consequences for individual range from none to severe. Symptoms can include vulvar pain, dyspareunia (painful sexual intercourse) and itching. In addition, there may be reduced lubrication [10] associated with sexual arousal and a reduction in vaginal blood flow and engorgement.

The clitoris diminishes in size and [11] vaginal penetration may be more difficult as the labia may not fully elevate; the vaginal barrel shortens and narrows and if present, the cervix may drop increasing the chance of cervical bumping. All these factors can influence penetrative sexual intercourse, but it is important to recognise many people have fully satisfactory sex lives without vaginal penetration. As woman age, vaginal contractions are fewer and weaker, but the orgasmic or multi-orgasmic response remains [10].

The impact of the menopause on sexual functioning may mean a reduction in the quality of sexual intercourse but should not impact on other sexual activity [12]. Regular pelvic floor exercises increase tone and reduce the risk of urinary incontinence and that hormone replacement therapy (HRT) may still be appropriate for some women, which may ameliorate some discomfort. There are many myths associated with the menopause but with good health, a good relationship and appropriate healthcare sexual vigour may continue in the mature years of a woman's life. We need to be conscious of an increasing "medicalisation" of sexual function with many treatments such as lubrication being available over the counter in pharmacies, supermarkets and over the Internet. There is an increased prevalence of both breast and endometrial cancer in older women, which have implications for body image, self-esteem and sexual response.

6.4.2 Changes in the Male Body

As men age, the reduction of testosterone may result in less rigid erections, weaker ejaculations, longer time to ejaculation; additionally, there is a decreased likelihood of orgasms and longer refractory periods. Meston [13] states, there is a decline in scrotal vasocongestion, reduced tensing of the scrotal sac and delayed erection.

The prevalence of prostatism also increases with age. Prostatism occurs when there is overgrowth of the prostate gland, which may be benign or malignant. The symptom of nocturia (passing urine at night and frequently associated with prostatism) is common; around one third of men will develop urinary tract (outflow) symptoms, all of which can have significant impact on sexual activity. Penile sensitivity also decreases with age and rates of impotence increase.

Impotence can cause psychological difficulties for men, leading to sexual avoidance and aversion; the nature of partner's responses to sexual problems is significant as lack of support can lead to further difficulties [14]. It is important to reflect that the research in this area has focussed on heterosexual couples.

6.4.3   Changes Concerning Both Sexes

It is acknowledged that where a decline in sexual activity occurs, this is usually due to age-associated change and reduction in mobility, although it must be stated that long-term conditions, such as diabetes, cardiovascular disease and cancer, can have a negative impact on sexual activity and that the prevalence of such conditions increases with age ([15].

Urinary incontinence can have considerable impact on older people's sexual activity due to its effects on self-esteem and on desire if one's partner experiences incontinence. Frequent causes are obesity, oestrogen depletion (in women), neurological conditions such as Parkinson's disease or multiple sclerosis, urinary tract infections and medication. Overflow incontinence is often caused by bladder obstruction, which may result from constipation or bladder stones, in men bladder obstruction may also be due to enlarged prostate.

In summary, physiological sexual changes occur for both men and women in older age, and these may impact on their previous choice of sexual function; however, such changes do not necessarily result in an inability to maintain sexual activity or even coitus. Good physical health and the ability to discuss issues are shown to help older people to remain sexually active. As health professionals caring for people with long-term conditions, our interactions offer an opportunity to discuss an individual's sexual health needs and help them plan for the future.

6.5   Barriers to Sexual Intimacy

Many older people received little or no formal sex education, growing up at a time when sexual behaviour was not discussed, and sexual feelings were suppressed. This was particularly true for women for whom sexual pleasure was not seen as being as important as procreation. Issues of non-binary sexuality were infrequently explored, and social influences of when sexual expression was appropriate and when it was not were strong. Homosexual activity was something that received both legal and moral sanction, and the ideas of being married and welcomed into mainstream community life may have been a far-off dream for many gay older people.

Reflective Questions
1. What are your views about sexual activity in older age?
   When you first decided to read this chapter, what were your initial thoughts?
2. Can you imagine if restrictions were placed on your current sexual activity or non-activity, simply because you aged?
   How would this make you feel?
   How would you challenge any restrictions?

6.5.1 Societal Barriers

In many societies, older people are often depicted as asexual beings, being seen as physically unattractive in a culture, which values youth [16]. However, these archaic stereotypes are beginning to change, with an emerging emphasis on sexuality through the life course [17]. Interestingly, this has brought with it or even occurred because of the medicalisation of sexual activity, with new pharmacological advances and an increased public awareness that the physiology of sexual activity can be maintained. Usually, this is seen through the prism of penile vaginal penetration as being the normative sexual activity. This approach can be problematic as it creates a "binary of functional versus dysfunctional and encourages a restriction of meaning and range in sexual expression". Carpenter's [2] life course work sets out an intersectionality framework, which acknowledges that both gender and sexual identity are entwined with other aspects of identity such as religion, disability and social class and result in the adoption of sexual beliefs and behaviours.

The current state of older relationships is diverse and changing. Later, life divorces and remarriage rates are steadily increasing, resulting in a more positive experience of older age for a number of people as previously older people may have felt compelled to remain in unsatisfactory relationships due to social mores. Conversely, some older people, notably gay people, are more likely to live alone [18] and may have the additional stressors of limited family support. Many older people who engage in new relationships have concerns about the effects on their wider families in practical and financial terms, and there has been little formal study on re-partnering later in life. However, for older heterosexual women particularly, there are concerns with the financial risk of entering into a relationship with a new man and in addition are fearful of a loss of autonomy. This fear can emerge from a time when men were seen to be the head of the household and controlled finances and expenditures. One of the major aspects to this disquiet is the fear of having to take on the role of "nurse" as a partner's health begins to deteriorate [19]. Also lacking is any cohesive national policy about older age sexual health needs. In the UK, policy documents under address the issues of sexuality and older people including the cultural changes that have been seen in the past 55 years associated with sexual behaviour.

Reflective Activity
Spend the next 24 hours observing the messages sent to citizens about sexual activity; these will often be implied or nuanced such as advertisements, music, social media product placement or in literature. Look at the value placed on aesthetic beauty, youth and fitness.

6.5.2   Stigma and Stereotypes

Older adults in western culture learn sex is for the young and beautiful. In older age, sex is shameful or non-existent, and this creates an internalised stigma and low self-esteem. Culturally, explicit depictions of sexualised older adults remain taboo. The media send clear cultural messages that sex is only for the young, and ageist beliefs endure despite improved understanding of sexuality and effective treatment for dysfunctions [6].

DeLamater [4] echoed the idea that physical changes should not affect the person's ability for sexual functioning (although it is acknowledged that changes may need to be made to accommodate the effects of ageing) and that the changes people experience are the result of social values. Clearly, a couple's attitudes to sexuality are an important influence on sexual behaviour. They view themselves in relation to the responses of wider society and that has a powerful influence on how they see themselves as sexual beings and is an important determinant in sexual activity. Despite societal discussion about sexuality, entrenched views of "normal behaviours" remain and if that means sex is for the young and stereotypically beautiful, it can have negative impact on how older people live their lives. However, as the population ages, we are beginning to see a demolition of the scripts (internalised cultural norms) that have shaped the discussions about and with older people's sexual activity, and this may be an even more profound change as the baby boomer generation ages further.

6.6   Barriers to Accessing Healthcare

We have long acknowledged that there is need for healthcare practitioners to undertake a holistic assessment, but there are a number of barriers to this. Dyer and Nair [20] suggest there are a wide range of reasons why nurses do not raise this issue, including a worry about causing offence, personal discomfort, concern about their own abilities and the range of issues, and that they might not consider it their responsibility.

Some nurses feel ill-equipped and may be too embarrassed to talk about sexual implications of medical conditions or treatment regimes. It is clear that the sexual needs of older people are rarely discussed in the pre-registration curriculum of any healthcare professionals [21]. For many older people, both the normal processes of ageing and the pathological changes, such as incontinence, erectile difficulties and painful sexual relations, go unresolved because they are unable to seek help. Physical access to sexual health clinics can be restrictive, particularly if the older person has mobility or transportation difficulties, or simply feels clinics are tailored for younger people. In fact, sexual health clinic can offer a wide range of information and advice for older people, particularly around sexually transmitted disease, and can consider whether psychosexual support might be needed. Additionally, older people could have conversations with members of a primary healthcare team. However, we know communication difficulties because of embarrassment may mean that older people who desire sexual intimacy but have health needs may keep this to themselves and not feel able to approach healthcare practitioners.

6.7 Enablers for Sexual Intimacy in Older Age

Older people have experienced many social changes. In the postmodern period, marriage was not a prerequisite to sex, and couples are increasingly able to make their own sexual rules. The increase in free choice also means that if relationships did not work, couples are no longer compelled to stay together. There is an increase in the possibilities for people to be intimate and relax, but paradoxically people's expectations of their partners had also risen, which may add pressure for individuals.

The technological advances, which have changed social activities, now include the development of Internet dating, which enables older people to seek different relationships to those that they have previously experienced [22], potentially allowing them to express different elements of their sexuality or engage in different roles. In addition to the Internet being used for dating, it can answer potentially awkward medical questions and provide new sexual information. Older people use the Internet to purchase sexual adjuncts, including medications purporting to be Viagra, engage with online chat rooms, pornography or request sexual services. This may afford new sexual freedoms but can bring additional issues and potential exploitation.

6.7.1 Relationships

Within older people's relationships, sexual intimacy can be a great joy and contribute to a sense of comfort and well-being. The current generation of older people in the UK have access to some of the best healthcare in the world and a good standard of living. Unlike their predecessors, they have long periods of retirement and frequently have the health, time and money to invest in their relationships. They have devised new models of living; bringing together of houses or apartments has resulted in different forms of cohabitation, sometimes referred to as "Living Apart Together", where older people perceive themselves as a couple, but for family or financial reasons choose to own or rent their own homes.

6.7.2 Information About Sexuality for Older People

There are now specific websites for older people and many self-help books available; the websites often suggest changing the type of sexual activity to non-penetrative sex, mutual masturbation, giving and receiving oral sex, promoting physical exercise and some educational information. There are a large number of Internet sites accessible, and healthcare practitioners should be aware of trusted sites that they can refer older people to; the resources section of this chapter offers a number of helpful sites.

6.7.3 Interventions

There are a number of medications, which can help facilitate sexual intimacy. Women are able to access hormone replacement therapy, for men the use of drugs in the phosphodicstcrase-5 enzyme inhibitors group (drugs which include Viagra) can sometimes be used if they are experiencing erectile dysfunction. These drugs do not cause erections but affect the response to sexual stimulation by increasing blood flow to the corpora cavernosa and corpora spongiosum by smooth muscle relaxation, enhancing erections. The widespread use of this drug and others in the group clearly demonstrates a need for such medication. Lubrication, both water-soluble and oestrogen-enhanced (for women), is now more readily available and frequently prescribed. As well as these medications, a more sophisticated use of analgesia, may also promote sexual activity by allaying pain [23].

This section has demonstrated that there is a range of interventions that support sexual intimacy, and the picture is likely to further develop over the coming years, but the evidence base is scant and the potential for enhancing sexual intimacy not fully understood.

6.8   The Role of Healthcare Practitioners

It is recognised that sexuality and sexual health needs are under-assessed components of healthcare practice. Many older people have said they had never had an opportunity to speak about sex before and would value the opportunity ([24]. Nurses are often the first healthcare professionals that patients talk to, and the attitudes and response of the nurse will affect such conversations. It is known that a nurse's discomfort with the subject may cause them to unconsciously limit their interaction that would otherwise promote a discussion of the person's sexual needs [25]. It is important that healthcare professionals acknowledge their difficulties about discussing sex and realise that we are all influenced by societal and cultural messages about sexuality. Clinical supervisions and case discussion can provide opportunities to explore our own beliefs and values about sexual intimacy and older people.

There are a number of issues we should all be able to provide advice and signposting about these include STIs. We know that older people are less likely to use condoms and that within the UK, the prevalence of STIs is increasing in later life [26], demonstrating a clear need for clinicians to address matters of sexuality with older people.

Healthcare professionals need to be aware that patients often use diagnostic terminology in imprecise ways. Whilst good history taking is important, Skultety [10] explains sexual discussion is less about the details and more about the beliefs and ideas relating to sexual activity. She states, it is crucial to allow and encourage a broad definition of and consider a range of sexual behaviours and not purely concentrate on sexual intercourse.

Some older people may have gender preferences and may be more comfortable talking about sex with someone of the same gender. There are many opportunities to bring up the topic of sexual intimacy in an easy and non-intrusive way. Such openings can be when discussing the effects of long-term conditions on health, or breathlessness or pain. During rehabilitation, the nurse can explain how mobility issues might be overcome to assist with physical positioning, and when discussing medication side effects, the effects on libido can introduce the subject. Similarly, we have mentioned the issues of incontinence, and this may also be an opportunity to talk about issues related to sexual intimacy. Many older people are just waiting for the opportunity or "permission" to discuss their sexual health needs. The conversations should be private and unhurried, and there may be need of opportunities built in for follow-up appointments or conversations.

6.8.1   The PLISSIT Model

There are some models and assessment tools for assisting healthcare practitioners in the recognition or treatment of sexual health needs. One of the most common models is the PLISSIT model of sex therapy, which sets out a therapeutic framework in which such issues can be discussed [27]. Obviously, sex therapy is a very specific skill and people should be referred for therapy, but the model is used in many settings and offers a method for introducing sexual health into clinical conversations.

PLISSIT has four levels of increasing intervention and interaction related to what kind of and how much help is given to a client. The varying levels largely revolve around what the client is looking for and how comfortable they are in discussing sexuality and sexual health.

The first level is *permission*, which involves the clinician giving the person permission to feel comfortable about a topic or permission to change their lifestyle or to get medical assistance. This level was created because many clients only require the permission to speak and voice their concerns about sexual issues in order to understand and move past them, often without needing the other levels of the model. The clinician, in acting as a receptive, non-judgmental listening partner, allows the client to discuss matters that would otherwise be too embarrassing for the individual to discuss.

The second level is *limited information*, wherein the client is supplied with limited and specific information on the topics of discussion. Because there is a significant amount of information available, healthcare professionals must learn what sexual topics the client wishes to discuss, so that information, organisations and support groups for those specific subjects can be provided.

The third level is *specific suggestions*, where the specialist gives the client suggestions related to the specific situations and assignments to do in order to help the client fix the mental or health problem. This can include suggestions on how to deal with sex-related diseases or information on how to better achieve sexual satisfaction by the client changing their sexual behaviour. The suggestions may be as simple as recommending exercise or can involve specific regimens of activity or medications.

The fourth and final level is *intensive therapy*, which has the clinician refer the client to other mental and medical health professionals that can help the client deal with the deeper, underlying issues and concerns being expressed. This level, with the onset of the Internet age, may also refer to a specialist suggesting professional online resources for the client to browse about their specific issue in a more private setting.

6.9 Summary of Main Points

This chapter has looked at the wide range of issues relating to ageing and sexual intimacy including the psychosocial, physical and societal aspects of sexual health-care. There has been an exploration of the roles and responsibilities of healthcare practitioners. It is clear the practitioner's knowledge, skills and attitudes are essential to delivering holistic care and an assessment, which does not make reference to sexual health needs, is not a complete assessment. Practitioners need to understand their own bias and assumptions around older people and sexual intimacy. Sometimes, this will include dealing with uncomfortable feelings before providing sexual healthcare, and practitioners should have the opportunity to receive clinical supervision and to explore their concerns in safe environment.

The key message is that we need to have professional conversations with older people about their sexual health needs and to act on those expressions of need by appropriate and sensitive education, information, interventions or referral. We have both a duty and responsibility to ensure older people sexual rights are respected, protected and fulfilled.

6.10 Suggested Reading and URLs

Age UK https://www.ageuk.org.uk/information-advice/health-wellbeing/relation-ships-family/sex-in-later-life/#
  NHS https://www.nhs.uk/live-well/sexual-health/sex-as-you-get-older/
  https://www.evidence.nhs.uk/search?q=sexual+health+and+older+people

References

1. Maslow AH (1943) A theory of human motivation. Psychol Rev 50:370–396
2. Carpenter LM (2016) Studying sexualities from a life course perspective. In: Delamater J, Plante RF (eds) Handbook of the sociology of sexualities. Springer, Switzerland, pp 65–89
3. Age UK (2015) Long term conditions briefing. Age UK, London
4. Delamater J (2012) Sexual expression in later life: a review and synthesis. J Sex Res 49(2):125–141
5. Kohlbacher F, Herstatt C (2011) The silver market phenomenon: marketing and innovation in the aging society, 2nd edn. Springer, Berlin

6. Weeks DJ (2002) Sex for the mature adult: health, self-esteem and countering ageist stereotypes. Sex Relationsh Ther 17(3):231–249
7. World Health Organisation (2002) Defining sexual health: report of a technical consultation on sexual health. WHO. http://www.who.int/reproductivehealth/topics/sexual_health/sh_definitions/en/. Accessed 2 June 2017
8. World Health Organisation (n.d.) Defining sexual health. http://www.who.int/reproductivehealth/topics/sexual_health/sh_definitions/en/. Accessed 6 Dec 2016
9. World Health Organisation (2015) Sexual health, human rights and the law. WHO. http://apps.who.int/iris/bitstream/10665/175556/1/9789241564984_eng.pdf. Accessed 7 Jan 2018
10. Skultety KM (2007) Addressing issues of sexuality with older couples. Generations 31(3):31–37
11. Pariser SF, Niedermier JA (1998) Sex and the mature woman. J Womens Health 7(7):849–859
12. Ambler DR, Bieber EJ, Diamond MP (2012) Sexual function in elderly women: a review of current literature. Rev Obstet Gynecol 5(1):16–27
13. Meston CM (1997) Aging and sexuality. West J Med 167(4):285–290
14. Li H, Gao T, Wang R (2016) The role of the sexual partner in managing erectile dysfunction. Nat Rev Urol 13:168–177
15. Zeiss AM, Kasl-Godley J (2001) Sexuality in older adults' relationships. Generations 25(2):18–25
16. Menard AD, Kleinplatz PJ, Rosen L, Lawless S, Paradis N, Campbell M, Huber JD (2015) Individual and relational contributors to optimal sexual experiences in older men and women. Sex & Relationsh Ther 30(1):78–93
17. Public Health England (2015) Taking a life-course approach to sexual and reproductive health. Public Health England, London
18. Age UK (2018) https://www.ageuk.org.uk/our-impact/policy-research/loneliness-research-and-resources/combating-loneliness-amongst-older-lgbt-people-a-case-study-of-the-sage-project-in-leeds/
19. Bildtgard T, Öberg P (2015) Time as a structuring condition behind new intimate relationships in later life. Ageing Soc 35(7):1505–1528
20. Dyer K, Nair R (2012) Why don't healthcare professionals talk about sex? A systematic review of recent qualitative studies conducted in the United Kingdom. J Sex Med 10:2658–2670
21. Evans DT (2013) Promoting sexual health and wellbeing: the role of the nurse. Nurs Standard 28(10):53–57
22. McWilliams S, Barrett AE (2014) Online dating in middle and later life: gendered expectations and experiences. J Fam Issues 35:182–129
23. Miller CA (2004) Nursing for wellness in older adults: theory and practice. Lippincott Williams & Wilkins, Philadelphia
24. Gott M, Hinchliff S (2003) How important is sex in later life? The views of older people. Soc Sci Med 56(8):1617–1628
25. Mueller IW (1997) Clinical savvy. Common questions about sex and sexuality in elders. Am J Nurs 97(7):61–64
26. Public Health England (2016) New STI diagnoses & rates by gender sexual risk and age group 2011-2015. Public Health England, London
27. Annon JS (1976) The PLISSIT model: A proposed conceptual scheme for the behavioral treatment of sexual problems. J Sex Educ Ther 2(1):1–15

The Frailty Approach: Rest-of-Life Care of the Older Person

7

John Alexander McKay

Contents

7.1 Learning Objectives

This chapter will enable you to:

- Approach the complexity of elderly frail patients with confidence
- Adopt a systematic approach to assessment of the older person
- Quickly gain an accurate picture of your patient and their needs, to enable care-planning

J. A. McKay (✉)
East Cheshire NHS Trust Frailty Team, Macclesfield District General Hospital, Macclesfield, Cheshire, UK
e-mail: john.mckay@nhs.net

© Springer Nature Switzerland AG 2021
W. McSherry et al. (eds.), *Understanding Ageing for Nurses and Therapists*, Perspectives in Nursing Management and Care for Older Adults,
https://doi.org/10.1007/978-3-030-40075-0_7

7.2 Introduction

This chapter will address the complexity of older people's presentations. To do this, Frailty will be clearly defined and its emergence as an important clinical syndrome and diagnosis explained. By illustrating a logical and evidenced approach, you will have the confidence to apply this knowledge, equipped with the skills you need to effectively support and manage the frail elderly patient. The Frailty Approach is appropriate to all settings, where the nurse, therapist, health or social care professional encounters the elderly patient, be it on the hospital ward, in the Emergency Department, the out-patient clinic, in nursing or residential homes, hospice or the patient's own home.

> **Reflective Exercise**
> - *Why do you think it is important to have a knowledge and understanding of Frailty and its impact on older people?*

7.2.1 A Frailty Approach

Every one of us has a life story, a context which helps us to appreciate, understand and engage with. This forms an important part of the comprehensive assessment of older people. My mum was a nurse in the new National Health Service (NHS), training in London from 1951 to 1954. She was a ward sister. She survived cancer in her 30s living to be 90. She had a long, testing decline and demise from dementia, spending six and a half years in a residential home. In that time, she spoke poems I never heard her say before. My dad, having been looked after all his life, became the main carer for my mum; he developed an acute leukaemia and died at the age 78.

My wife is a nurse, my daughter is a nurse. My second daughter is training to be a speech and language therapist, my third daughter wants to be a social worker. My niece is a physiotherapist, currently recovering from coronavirus.

> **Reflective Exercise**
> - *What do you think are the types of conditions you will face when caring for frail older people?*
> - *What types of knowledge, skills, attitudes and behaviours do you need to do this compassionately and professionally?*
> - *'One of the essential qualities of the clinician is interest in humanity, for the secret of the care of the patient is in caring for the patient'* [1, p. 882]. *What do you think of this statement?*
> - *What is it that motivates and inspires you?*

This chapter is about rest-of-life care, a concept suggested to me by Elaine Horgan, an NHS manager in 2001. Rather than use 'end-of-life', she encouraged me to use the term 'rest-of-life'. This has since had a beneficial effect on the quality of conversations with relatives, patients and colleagues. The use of positive language, which was not immediately difficult for patients talking about 'the end', helped me and my patients and their relatives to talk about what is to come—'the rest of your life', a less threatening idea. Having been an NHS General Practitioner (GP) for 25 years, working in Care Homes for 15 years, General Practice and the local hospice, this chapter flows from the past 5 years in a hospital Frailty team. Our multidisciplinary team (MDT) approach uses the principles of Comprehensive Geriatric Assessment (CGA). CGA is 'a multidimensional, interdisciplinary diagnostic process to determine the medical, psychological and functional capabilities of a frail older person in order to develop a coordinated and integrated plan for treatment and long-term follow-up' [2]. Patricia Cantley's [3] paper boat on the pond illustrates well the concept of Frailty. An origami paper boat floating on a calm pond on a summer's day only betrays its Frailty when the sun retreats, the wind blows, and the boat is inundated with waves and eventually sinks. With good weather and gentle winds, the future for the paper boat can be good depending on prevailing conditions encountered. Such is the frail patient who is managed well with good care addressing challenges to their health. However, if the storms such as infection or falls strike, the patient's condition can become unsustainable.

Frailty is not new but, like Dementia, has become an important concept because of the non-specific nature of elderly presentations. The increasing number of older people requiring care is sometimes referred to as 'the Silver Tsunami' [4].

The demography of the challenge faced by health and care services will now be considered.

7.2.2 Demography: National and International

The population statistics below (Table 7.1) indicate that many people in specific parts of the world are living longer.

Table 7.1 Population statistics, World, Europe/North America and United Kingdom (UK) [5, 6]

World				
Over 65s		*Over 80s*		
2019 1 in 11 (9%)		143 million		
2050 1 in 6 (16%)		426 million		
Europe and North America				
Over 65s				
2050 1 in 4				
UK				
2019	>65 12 million >75 5.4 million	>85 1.6 million	>90 0.5 million	>100. 15,000
2030				>100. 21,000
2041		>85 3.2 million		
2066.		>85 5.1 million		

All health systems are serving ageing populations. The United Nations [6] states:

Globally, the population aged 65 and over is growing faster than all other age groups. In 2018, for the first time in history, persons aged 65 or above outnumbered children under five years of age globally.

In the UK [5], the 85+ age group is the fastest growing and is set to double to 3.2 million by mid-2041 and treble by 2066. Substantial progress has been made to enable people to live to a great age. However, health and social care systems need to be equipped to care for more people living for longer periods with progressive disability, dementia and Frailty. We will now consider the key elements of a Frailty Approach.

7.3   The Key Elements of a Frailty Approach: Defining the Core Concepts

This section will define and explain the core concepts including Frailty, Dementia, Delirium, Co-morbidity, Polypharmacy and Falls. They are foundational to an understanding of effective care of the elderly and relevant to all professionals involved.

7.3.1   Frailty: Definition of a Diagnosis

Frailty becomes more prevalent the older we become and is higher in the over 85s (Table 7.2).

Clegg et al. [8, p. 752] described Frailty as 'the most problematic expression of population ageing'. Rockwood et al. [9] described Frailty as a clinically valid and valuable concept, however, a difficult term to define well. Moody [10] defined Frailty as 'reduced resilience and increased vulnerability to decompensation after a stressor event'. The British Geriatric Society [11, p. 6] defines Frailty as:

a distinctive health state related to the ageing process in which multiple body systems gradually lose their in-built reserves.

Rockwood et al. [9] have described a practical, usable and reproducible 'deficit accumulation model' of Frailty, which says that 'small age-related problems add up to give rise to Frailty' [12]. The clinical frailty scale was developed (Fig. 7.1). It is popular in clinical practice today and has gained widespread recognition because it relies on professional judgement. It is used in many settings to screen for Frailty. It is

Table 7.2 Prevalence of frailty and age (adapted from British Geriatric Society, [7])

Age groups	Prevalence %
>65 years	10
>85 years	25–50

CLINICAL FRAILTY SCALE

	1	**VERY FIT**	People who are robust, active, energetic and motivated. They tend to exercise regularly and are among the fittest for their age.
	2	**FIT**	People who have **no active disease symptoms** but are less fit than category 1. Often, they exercise or are very **active occasionally**, e.g., seasonally.
	3	**MANAGING WELL**	People whose **medical problems are well controlled**, even if occasionally symptomatic, but often are **not regularly active** beyond routine walking.
	4	**LIVING WITH VERY MILD FRAILTY**	Previously "vulnerable," this category marks early transition from complete independence. While **not dependent on** others for daily help, often **symptoms limit activities.** A common complaint is being "slowed up" and/or being tired during the day.
	5	**LIVING WITH MILD FRAILTY**	People who often have **more evident slowing, and need help with high order instrumental activities of daily** living (finances, transportation, heavy housework). Typically, mild frailty progressively impairs shopping and walking outside alone, meal preparation, medications and begins to restrict light housework.
	6	**LIVING WITH MODERATE FRAILTY**	People who need help with **all outside activities** and with **keeping house.** Inside, they often have problems with stairs and need **help with bathing** and might need minimal assistance (cuing, standby) with dressing.
	7	**LIVING WITH SEVERE FRAILTY**	**Completely dependent for personal care**, from whatever cause (physical or cognitive). Even so, they seem stable and not at high risk of dying (within ~6 months).
	8	**LIVING WITH VERY SEVERE FRAILTY**	Completely dependent for personal care and approaching end of life. Typically, they could not recover even from a minor illness.
	9	**TERMINALLY ILL**	Approaching the end of life. This category applies to people with a **life expectancy <6 months**, who are **not otherwise living with severe frailty.** (Many terminally ill people can still exercise until very close to death.)

SCORING FRAILTY IN PEOPLE WITH DEMENTIA

The degree of frailty generally corresponds to the degree of dementia. Common **symptoms in mild dementia** include forgetting the details of a recent event, though still remembering the event itself, repeating the same question/story and social withdrawal.

In **moderate dementia**, recent memory is very impaired, even though they seemingly can remember their past life events well. They can do personal care with prompting.

In **severe dementia**, they cannot do personal care without help.

In **very severe dementia** they are often bedfast. Many are virtually mute.

DALHOUSIE UNIVERSITY
www.geriatricmedicineresearch.ca

Clinical Frailty Scale ©2005–2020 Rockwood, Version 2.0 (EN). All rights reserved. For permission: www.geriatricmedicineresearch.ca Rockwood K et al. A global clinical measure of fitness and frailty in elderly people. CMAJ 2005;173:489–495.

Fig. 7.1 The Clinical Frailty Scale (CFS) version 2.0. With permission from Dalhousie University, Geriatric Medicine Research

relevant for health professionals because it provides shareable information. Rockwood [13] wrote: '[it gives] information from a clinical encounter with an older person, [to] roughly quantify an individual's overall health status'. It is this description which is useful and shareable for all health and social care professionals.

7.3.2 Dementia and Its Close Connection with Frailty

A 2020 UK National Institute for Health and Care Excellence [14] dementia impact report shows that approximately 460,000 people in England are diagnosed with dementia, and a further 200,000 are estimated to be undiagnosed.

Dementia is an umbrella term used to describe a range of progressive neurological disorders, conditions affecting the brain. There are over 200 subtypes of dementia, but the five most common are: Alzheimer's disease, vascular dementia, dementia with Lewy bodies, frontotemporal dementia and mixed dementia. Mixed dementia is a combination of different types. [15, p. 2].

Dementia contributes to Frailty by damaging brain cells and preventing the brain from functioning normally.

It is estimated that 25% of hospital beds are occupied by someone with dementia. However, the Alzheimer's Society estimates that this is a very low estimate and states that the figure is far more likely to be as high as 50% [16].

7.3.3 Delirium

This next section introduces you to an important condition that is often overlooked or under-diagnosed when caring for older people

> Delirium (or "acute confusional state") is a common clinical syndrome characterised by disturbed consciousness, cognitive function or perception, which has an acute onset and fluctuating course. It usually develops over 1–2 days [17].

Delirium can be defined as any acute change in normal cognitive state. It can be either hyperactive (restless, agitated with poor concentration) or hypoactive (withdrawn, quiet and sleepy) [18]. Delirium is important because it is a serious condition associated with poor outcomes. However, it can be prevented and treated if dealt with urgently [17].

The causes of both hypo and hyperactive delirium are the same [18]. See Fig. 7.2 below [19].

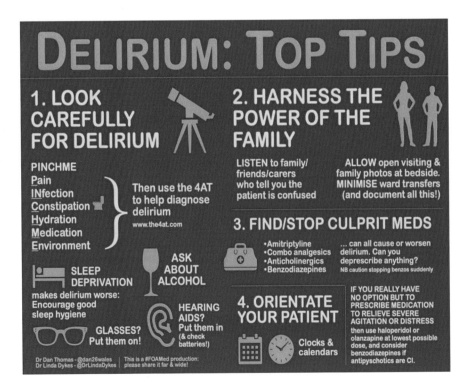

Fig. 7.2 Delirium: top tips with permission of Dr Daniel Thomas and Dr Linda Dykes ©Dr Linda Dykes and Dr Daniel Thomas

A good place to start with delirium is to ask a relative or carer the 'single question to identify delirium', the SQuID [20]. 'Is the patient more confused than normal?' Then the Abbreviated Mental Test (AMT4), a four-question test, is used. It consists of asking place, age, date of birth and current year. It is simple, quick and easy to administer:

> *The way to propose it to the patient to minimise anxiety is not to start straight in with the questions otherwise they may feel you are trying to catch them out or lay bare their deficiencies. Rather, begin with the question 'How do you feel about your memory?', then ask: 'Would you mind if I ask you 4 quick questions'. Having been asked in such a careful and respectful manner, the patient almost never objects. It is invaluable to be able quickly establish the presence or absence of cognitive impairment in your first moments of assessment.*

The AMT4 is a validated rapid initial cognitive estimate. 'Using a four-question test to determine a patient's cognitive functioning is very useful since time pressure is at the heart of making a comprehensive enough assessment' [21]. Importantly, many patients have delirium against a background of dementia. Some have delirium only without any associated or diagnosed dementia. The important thing to remember is that with delirium it is of **recent and rapid onset.**

7.3.4 Perplexing Behaviour

Delirium and dementia are often characterised by behavioural and psychological symptoms. This is often referred to as challenging behaviour or behaviours that challenge to try to reduce stigma. A better term is perplexing behaviour—which is non-stigmatising, and it states the reality—it is perplexing for patient, carers and health professionals.

7.3.5 Capacity

The main principle here is to ensure that the system acts in the best interests of the patient, which relates to the Mental Capacity Act of 2005. Assessing capacity causes difficulties for health and care professionals.

Assessing capacity needs a consideration of four things:

1. Understanding
2. Retention
3. Evaluation
4. Communication

Capacity assessment involves decision-making such as resuscitation status and preferred place of care when the patient is not able to decide. A patient may be able to decide what they would like for lunch but not have capacity to consent to treatment. Consultation with relatives is important. Remember capacity is decision-specific. Capacity is associated with Powers of Attorney and Deprivation of Liberty. These are referred to in the further learning section.

7.3.6 Polypharmacy: How Medications Can Cause Rather Than Solve Problems

Polypharmacy literally means multiple medicines. The National Service Framework of 2001 established the need for 'discontinuing inappropriate or excessive medication' [22]. Polypharmacy can be either appropriate or inappropriate. Polypharmacy increases the risk and predisposition of falls. Older people are more susceptible to side effects, which can lead to falls. A useful mnemonic is CAPTAIN—Check All Prescribing To Ascertain If Needed. Rationalising medication with appropriate deprescribing should be the norm. If you see a lengthy list of medications, approach a colleague who can review this. This will usually be a doctor or pharmacist. More nurses and allied health professionals are becoming prescribers. Regular medication review is crucial in older people, especially in falls and treating delirium. There are guidelines which encourage health and care professionals to think carefully about medications and their unwanted effects. For example, the STOPP/START criteria [23].

Frailty, delirium, dementia, medication side effects and falls are the main problems encountered in caring for older people. Depression is also a problem in old age; however, side effects of antidepressants particularly increased falls risk must be considered. Antidepressants increase falls risk through exacerbating postural drops in BP and slowing response time [24]. The measurement of lying and standing blood pressure to detect postural drops is mandatory in all fallers [25].

7.3.7 Co-morbidities

Co-morbidity or multi-morbidity (the presence of multiple co-morbidities) refers to having two or more long-term physical or mental health conditions [26]. Many of our older people have multiple co-morbidities resulting in cumulative deficits. These deficits can be physical, social, functional and cognitive. For example, one older person could have the following co-morbidities: dementia, diabetes, Frailty and chronic obstructive pulmonary disease (COPD). Multimorbidity results in cumulative deficits.

7.3.8 Falls

Falls happen when Frailty, delirium, dementia, polypharmacy and co-morbidities conspire together.

> Falls remain a major cause of injury and death amongst the over 70s and account for more than 50 per cent of hospital admissions for accidental injury [27].

Medications can contribute to the risk of falling such as those used to control blood pressure, diabetes, angina, heart disease, depression, anxiety, enlarged prostate, strong pain killers and sleeping tablets [24].

Everyone who falls should have a lying and standing blood pressure, this is something which is often omitted and, therefore, postural drops missed.

7.3.9 Deconditioning

Muscle loss associated with prolonged stays in bed prejudices recovery. Anti-deconditioning campaigns have become prominent in the UK in an attempt to combat this. The importance of early mobilisation, where possible, encouraged by dressing patients in their own clothes is clear. Initiatives such as 'End PJ Paralysis' [28] have been introduced. Patients look so much healthier when dressed in their own clothes, and this approach is to be encouraged. It fits well with CGA.

7.4 Comprehensive Geriatric Assessment: Crossing Boundaries Not Patrolling Them

We have looked at the key concepts around care of the older person. These concepts now come together as they combine into the tool called CGA, which will equip you with the skills you need to undertake assessment and treatment of the older person with confidence, whether your core expertise is social care, nursing, therapy or medicine.

Crossing Professional and Practical Boundaries Not Patrolling Them: A Frailty team is part of everyone's team looking to interact with all professionals involved in a person's care. An 'approach' is the way we assess and build a picture of the patient. Engaging with patients is always time-pressured in whatever setting you find yourself, hence the emphasis is on a 'comprehensive enough' assessment.

7.4.1 Comprehensive Geriatric Assessment: A Proven Tool

Frail older patients often present in a non-specific way with one or more of the 5 Is: *instability (falls), immobility, iatrogenic presentations (polypharmacy), impairment of cognition and incontinence* [29].

CGA is a tool which is aimed at breaking down the complexity of the presentations of older people into manageable chunks. It is accessible to all health and care professionals and depends on contributions from all professionals involved. All of their core skills create an accurate and shareable picture of the patient's presentation. Too often, different caring professions complete their tasks in isolation. This is a way of integrating health and social care assessment in a constructive and beneficial way. It benefits the professionals involved by encouraging dialogue. The fact these professionals work in the same team means they are easily accessible to each other. A practical and helpful definition describes CGA as:

A process of good, holistic care delivered within a geriatric-medicine-focused multi-disciplinary team, which goes above and beyond simply managing the acute problem that the person has presented with' [30].

The evidence for the success of CGA is threefold:

1. It leads to better outcomes than 'usual medical care' (going beyond addressing just the problem the patient presented with, for example, pneumonia)
2. CGA makes people more likely to be alive in a year and to be living a less-dependent life.
3. It has been so successful that it is being used in other disciplines [30].

Recent developments have seen it used to assess patients following fractures (ortho-geriatrics) and in cancer patients (oncogeriatrics). It is also being used to assess patients, where surgery is being considered (POPS: Preoperative pre-surgical assessment). CGA needs the skills of all the multidisciplinary team, that is, all the caring professions, otherwise it loses its benefits [30].

7.4.2 The Four Domains of the CGA: MSFC—Medical, Social, Functional and Cognitive

Assessment takes time but can be done initially rapidly and can be repeated going deeper each time.

- *Quick example of the usefulness of CGA—86 years patient comes in—witnessed fall, from a Care home, reduced mobility. Medical—Fall, Social—Residential Home, Function—wheeled Zimmer Frame, Cognition—Known dementia. Immediately the goal of care will be to return this patient to their Residential home once their appropriate investigations have been completed, including medication review (CAPTAIN), bloods and x-rays, discussion with carers, mobility assessment and assessment of cognition. Lying and standing blood pressure checked once fractures excluded—LSBPCOFE!*

7.4.2.1 Medical: A Foundation But Only 25% of the Story

The medical domain of a CGA must include the presenting problem, past medical history and the current medication of the patient as well as allergies. It is an important part of the assessment but is only 25% of it. The social, functional and cognitive aspects remain essential to the patient's progress. In drawing together the medical element of a CGA, use can be made of the following sources: general practitioner (GP) computer systems, social care records, phoning local social services, paramedic admission sheets, GP admission letters and emergency department (ED) letters.

7.4.2.2 Social: The Context of Day-to-Day Living

The social domain must include significant others, care packages and agency contact numbers. This part is about recruiting allies for the ongoing care of the patient outside of hospital. Communication and consultation with relatives and carers has helped me greatly in my practice in terms of accurate history and planning future care.

It is important to engage the skills and knowledge of local social care professionals as early as possible as they know how to navigate the often-confusing array of care providers and funding issues.

7.4.2.3 Functional: The Importance of the Multidisciplinary Approach

This domain includes home layout including stairs, toilet and washing provision, whether upstairs or downstairs, activities of daily living (ADLs) and mobility assessment, use of walking aids such as Zimmer frames and continence.

One of the key tenets of CGA is the skills of therapists, particularly physiotherapists and occupational therapists. The importance of optimising mobility and dealing with environmental considerations is crucial.

7.4.2.4 Cognition: Rapid But Accurate

Impaired cognition brought by impaired vision and hearing is identified—poor sight and hearing should be recorded, and hearing aids and glasses found. Cognition can be assessed with the AMT4 and SQuID (single question to identify delirium): 'Is this person more confused than before?' The AMT4 can be supplemented later in the patient journey by the 4AT delirium screen.

7.4.2.5 Summarising: Recording and Making a Plan of Care

A CGA can be simply summarised under the four headings: medical, social, functional and cognitive problems leading to a plan of goals. Admission or discharge of the patient into the appropriate clinical setting is guided by the CGA. CGA is not a once-and-for-ever event. It is used as the repeated way of processing the current presentation of the patient to inform ongoing and future care.

7.5 Practical Application of CGA: A Clinical Scenario Employing Tips and Tools Described in This Chapter

Case:

Violet is 92 and lives alone. She is admitted to the ED after being found on the floor at home by the 9 a.m. carer. No active bleeding, she has been conveyed by the ambulance service because of left hip pain. Violet has dementia—confusion suddenly worse in last 2 days according to carer. She is on 12 different medications.

Reflective Exercise:
Initial Consideration of the Following

- **Which of the 5 Is is Violet presenting with?**
  1. **Immobility:** Yes, currently, what is her normal baseline mobility?
  2. **Instability:** Yes
  3. **Iatrogenic:** Yes, probable polypharmacy—12 medications
  4. **Incontinence:** Perhaps—check with the carers.
  5. **Impairment of cognition:** Do the SQuID and AMT4—place, age, DOB, year (PADY)
- **What are her medical problems (include consideration of the possible harmful effects of medications)?**
- **What are her social problems?**
- **What are her functional problems?**
- **What are her cognitive problems?**

- *Document sources of your information with contact numbers—it will help you later. Next consider the problems Violet presents under the following headings:*
  - *Medical Problems*: Initial assessment to exclude sepsis. Fall, polypharmacy, Frailty (Rockwood level—6)—consult computerised and paper records. Lying and standing blood pressure required, given the fall and polypharmacy (Defer until hip fracture has been excluded but ensure requirement recorded in notes as a reminder to self and colleagues). Ensure appropriate assessment by medical colleague with documented BP, pulse regular/irregular, temperature, oxygen saturation and appropriate blood samples. Imaging of left hip. Violet also needs a computer tomography (CT) of her brain because she is taking an oral anticoagulant for atrial fibrillation and, therefore, may have had an intra-cerebral bleed [31]. Her worsened confusion could be compounded by a head injury.
  - *Social Problems*: **Does she live in a house/flat or care home? Has she got family? Enlist their support. Ring them if not present. Are they coping? Does she have a package of care?**
  - Package of care in place for the last 3 years (information from social services as care agency unavailable. Also give your daughter's contact number).
  - Next of kin is a daughter who lives 200 miles away, she comes infrequently and does weekly food shopping online. House with stairs. Widow for 10 years.
  - *Functional*: **Consider ADLs, mobility, use of aids and continence. Consider the environment—stairs? Where does she sleep? Where is the loo –upstairs or downstairs?**
  - Violet lives downstairs with a commode for toileting as she can no longer manage the stairs and no downstairs loo. She uses a Zimmer frame and is unsteady on her feet (information from daughter by phone). She is incontinent of urine with occasional faecal incontinence. Pads from bowel and bladder service.

- *Cognitive*: **Use a quickly administrable and recordable AMT4: place, age, DOB, year and record the score. Presence or absence of cognitive deficit is an important initial feature to capture by also using the SQuID.**
- The SQuID: 'Is the patient's confusion worse than normal?' Care Agency Golden Days 9 a.m. carer confirmed to daughter that Violet has been more agitated and anxious in last 2 days. Violet scores 1 out of 4 on the AMT4—place x, age x, DOB correct, year x.

- *How would you summarise your information, record it and establish the overall goal of this episode? To whom would you refer the patient?*

This information is recorded under the four headings:

- **Medical**: moderately frail lady of 92 years, background of hypertension, vascular dementia, previous stroke, carcinoma of breast 15 years ago. Fall possible head injury. Increased confusion/agitation for 2 days.
- Rockwood Clinical frailty scale—6.
- **Social**: Package of Care Golden Days agency 01625 444 323, 3 × daily.
- Daughter Fiona, London. 020 7345 2001. Online shopping. Visits fortnightly.
- Neighbours 'look in.' Suggests patient vulnerable overnight.
- **Function**: House with stairs. Downstairs living, Zimmer frame, unsteady, fall 3 months ago
- Baseline: able to stand independently and transfer
- Incontinent of urine, occasional faecal incontinence, pads from bladder/bowel service
- **Cognition**: AMT4 1/4 Hearing aids—left at home, poor sight. Known dementia

Plan
- Get hearing aids and glasses from home
- Refer to orthopaedics (bone fracture specialists)—confirmed L fracture neck of femur on X-ray
- Computerised tomography Brain scan—no bleeding identified
- Lying/standing blood pressure later because of fracture. Medicines optimisation (note Violet is on 12 medications)
- Needs deprivation of liberty safeguard as lacks capacity to consent to treatment currently
- May require intermediate (step down) care and then possible nursing home placement. Dr Jones has mentioned discussion of resuscitation status with daughter Fiona because of advancing Frailty and co-morbidities. For further discussion if condition worsens. Violet unable to engage with discussion. Daughter has Power of Attorney for Health and Wealth.
- From discussion with Violet's daughter, preferred place of care is home
- Handover to orthopaedic ward completed

Having looked at a clinical scenario, which demonstrates CGA in action, further areas for consideration going deeper are suggested next.

7.6   Summary

This chapter demonstrates the complex and often non-specific nature of older people's presentations clearly describing a tool to break that complexity down into
manageable 'bite-size' pieces. That tool is CGA. The value of CGA is shown. It
integrates the input of all the care professionals involved. Frail elderly people
require care beyond purely medical considerations. CGA also describes patients'
social, functional and cognitive problems—a Frailty Approach.

The key elements of a Frailty approach are described. The value of being able to
quantify an older person's overall health status and be able to share that information
with colleagues [13] is explained. The essential nature of an MDT approach is also
explained. How that approach considers the key concepts of dementia, delirium and
polypharmacy is described.

The CAPTAIN maxim is introduced—'Check All Prescribing To Ascertain If
Needed'. The burden of falls and their incidence and causes, often related to polypharmacy, is described, along with the importance of ensuring every faller has a
lying and standing blood pressure recorded and evaluated.

Having described the Frailty team and its ability to challenge traditional care
boundaries and roles, its main tool CGA is outlined with its proven benefits of
improving survival and keeping people in their own homes. The four domains of
CGA are then described in detail. How medical, social, functional and cognitive
problems contribute to overall health status is demonstrated, with clear care planning made possible. The scenario of 92-year-old Violet's presentation to hospital
shows how the principles described are applied in practice.

Further learning opportunities are described below with information about the
people and organisations making a difference to the care of older people.

I would like to acknowledge the dedication and support of my colleagues in the
Frailty team at Macclesfield hospital as well as Sian Harrison, Cheshire Advanced
Dementia Team for help with Demography, Dr. Dawn Moody for the term 'Frailty
Approach' and Elaine Horgan, NHS Manager for the term 'rest-of-life'.

7.7   Taking It Further: Suggested Further Reading

MDTea Podcasts. 'The MDTea is a project with an interest in podcasts and the
power of storytelling. A suite of resources for those health and social care professionals that are lucky enough to work with older people'. http://thehearingaidpod-
casts.org.uk/about/

The British Geriatric Society—all things relevant to older people's care.
bgs.org.uk

Dawn Moody, Former Deputy National Director for Older People at NHS England, has created resources to benefit patient management, for example, the Virtual
Reality Frailty experience along with the Frailty toolkit: https://www.frailtytoolkit.
org/frailty360-intro/

Ethics of care—the 4 principles of Respect for Autonomy, Beneficence, Non-
maleficence and Justice. Useful guide to ethical care when facing the dilemmas

posed by elderly patients. Tom Beauchamp and James Childress, *Principles of biomedical ethics*, 8th Edition, Oxford University Press, New York, January 2019.

End of Life issues. The Cheshire Advanced Dementia Support Team aims to guide and educate professionals and informal caregivers. http://eolp.co.uk/advanced-dementia-support-team/. The Gold Standards Framework led by Professor Keri Thomas. https://www.goldstandardsframework.org.uk

Dementia Friends run by the Alzheimer's Society—Accessible to all community groups for free. https://www.alzheimers.org.uk/get-involved/dementia-friendly- communities/dementia-friends

Admiral nurses—Dementia UK—the work of specialist dementia nurses. https://www.dementiauk.org/?gclid=CjwKCAjw2a32BRBXEiwAUcugiE-1nho4euQJDyeEnTQo9gb6OSlfJJv08MK8AvPfriHlXhsHp_RfehoC0Q0QAvD_BwE

Power of Attorney—Age UK, (2019), *Making sure your wishes are respected* https://www.ageuk.org.uk/globalassets/age-uk/documents/information-guides/ageukig21_powers_of_attorney_inf.pdf

DoLS—Lorraine Curry, (2017), *Quick Guide to Deprivation of liberty Safeguards* https://www.adass.org.uk/media/5896/quick-guide-to-deprivation-of-liberty-safeguards.pdf (DoLS).

References

1. Peabody FW (1927) The care of the patient. JAMA 88:876–882. https://depts.washington.edu/medhmc/wordpress/wp-content/uploads/Peabody.html. Accessed 28 June 2020
2. Roberts H, Conroy S (2018) Hospital wide CGA. https://www.bgs.org.uk/resources/hospital-wide-comprehensive-geriatric-assessment-how-cga-history-of-the-project. Accessed 27 Mar 2020
3. Patricia Cantley (2018) The Paper Boat. British Geriatric Society. https://www.bgs.org.uk/blog/the-paper-boat. Accessed 25 May 2020
4. Weinstein S (2015, April 2) The 'Silver Tsunami', Choosing how and where we age. [Web log post] https://www.psychologytoday.com/blog/what-do-i-do-now/201504/the-silver-tsunami. Accessed 1 Mar 2020
5. Age UK (2019) Later Life in the United Kingdom 2019. https://www.ageuk.org.uk/globalassets/age-uk/documents/reports-and-publications/later_life_uk_factsheet.pdf. Accessed 20 Mar 2020
6. United Nations (2019) Ageing, trends in population ageing. World population prospects: the 2019 revision. https://www.un.org/en/sections/issues-depth/ageing/. Accessed 20 Mar 2020
7. British Geriatric Society (2014) Fit for frailty. https://www.bgs.org.uk/resources/resource-series/fit-for-frailty. Accessed 24 June 2019
8. Clegg A, Young J, Iliffe S, Rikkert MO, Rockwood K (2013) Frailty in elderly people. Lancet 381(9868):752–762
9. Rockwood K, Song X, MacKnight C, Bergman H, Hogan DB, McDowell I, Mitnitski A (2005) A global clinical measure of fitness and frailty in elderly people. CMAJ 173(5):489–495. https://doi.org/10.1503/cmaj.050051
10. Moody D (2016) Identifying and understanding frailty. The North East Frailty Summit 5th Dec 2016. http://old.ahsn-nenc.org.uk/wpcontent/uploads/2016/11/Dawn-Moody.pdf. Accessed 6 Jan 2020
11. British Geriatric Society (2014) Gill Turner, Fit for Frailty Part 1, Consensus best practice guidance for the care of older people living in the community and outpatient settings. A report by the British Geriatrics Society in association with the Royal College of General

Practitioners and Age UK, p 6. https://www.bgs.org.uk/sites/default/files/content/resources/files/2018-05-23/fff_full.pdf. Accessed 24 June 2019

12. Rockwood et al (2020) Geriatric medicine research, our work on frailty and deficit accumulation. Dalhousie University, Halifax, Nova Scotia, Canada. https://www.dal.ca/sites/gmr/our-work.html. Accessed 27 Mar 2020

13. Rockwood et al (2020) Geriatric medicine research, our tools. https://www.dal.ca/sites/gmr/our-tools/clinical-frailty-scale.html (Permission for use granted https://www.dal.ca/sites/gmr/our-tools/permission-for-use.html). Dalhousie University, Halifax, Nova Scotia, Canada. Accessed 23 Mar 2020

14. National Institute for Health and Care Excellence (2020) Impact Dementia. https://www.nice.org.uk/about/what-we-do/into-practice/measuring-the-use-of-nice-guidance/impact-of-our-guidance/niceimpact-dementia. Accessed 30 Mar 2020

15. Dementia UK (2020) Understanding dementia, what is dementia? https://www.dementiauk.org/get-support/diagnosis-and-next-steps/what-is-dementia/. Accessed 30 Mar 2020

16. Alzheimer's Society (2016) Fix dementia care: hospitals, p 10

17. National Institute for Health and Care Excellence (2010) Delirium: prevention, diagnosis and management Clinical guideline [CG103]. Last updated: 14 Mar 2019. https://www.nice.org.uk/guidance/cg103/chapter/Introduction. Accessed 22 May 2020

18. Preston J, Wilkinson I (2016) The hearing aid podcasts - episode 1.2 delirium. http://thehearingaidpodcasts.org.uk/episode-1-2-delirium/. Accessed 22 May 2020

19. Thomas D, Wykes L (2018) Delirium infographic PINCHME. Delirium: top tips. https://www.lindadykes.org/infographics. Accessed 1 June 2020

20. Han JH, Schnelle JF, Wesley Ely E, Wilson A, Dittus RS (2018) An evaluation of single question delirium screening tools in older emergency department patients. Am J Emerg Med 36(7):1249–1252. in White KL (2019) Screening methods to identify delirium in the Emergency department. Masters in Geriatric Medicine, University of Salford, p 32

21. White KL (2019) Screening methods to identify delirium in the Emergency department. Masters in Geriatric Medicine, University of Salford, p 44

22. Department of Health. National Service Framework for older people, standard 6: Falls, p 80. https://assets.publishing.service.gov.uk/government/uploads/system/uploads/attachment_data/file/198033/National_Service_Framework_for_Older_People.pdf. Accessed 24 June 2019

23. O'Mahony D et al (2015) STOPP/START criteria for potentially inappropriate prescribing in older people: version 2. https://academic.oup.com/ageing/article/44/2/213/2812233. Accessed 24 June 2019

24. Darowski A (2008) Falls the facts. OUP, Oxford, p 67

25. Royal College of Physicians (2017) Measurement of lying and standing blood pressure: a brief guide for clinical staff. https://www.rcplondon.ac.uk/projects/outputs/measurement-lying-and-standing-blood-pressure-brief-guide-clinical-staff. Accessed 16 Jan 2020

26. National Institute for Health and Care Excellence (NICE) (2016) Multimorbidity: clinical assessment and management. NICE guideline [NG56]. https://www.nice.org.uk/guidance/NG56/chapter/Recommendations#multimorbidity. Accessed 24 June 2019

27. Age UK (2010) Falls in the over 65s cost NHS £4.6 million a day. https://www.ageuk.org.uk/latestpress/archive/falls-over-65s-cost-nhs/. Accessed 24 June 2019

28. NHS England (2018) EndPJParalysis: the revolutionary movement helping frail older people. https://www.england.nhs.uk/2018/06/endpjparalysis-revolutionary-movement-helping-frail-older-people/. Accessed 28 June 2020

29. Morley JE (2017) The new geriatric giants. https://www.geriatric.theclinics.com/article/S0749-0690(17)30037-X/fulltext. Accessed 21 Jan 2020

30. Preston J, Wilkinson I (2016) The hearing aid podcasts - Episode 1.1 comprehensive geriatric assessment. http://thehearingaidpodcasts.org.uk/episode-1-1-comprehensive-geriatric-assessment/#. Accessed 22 Mar 2020

31. National Institute for Health and Care Excellence (NICE) (2019) Triage, assessment, investigation and early management of head injury in infants, children and adults. https://www.nice.org.uk/guidance/cg176/chapter/1-recommendations

Nutrition and Ageing

8

Stacey Jones

Contents

8.1 Learning Objectives

This chapter will enable you to:

- Increase your knowledge of nutritional requirements for older people and recommendations for eating well for healthy ageing
- Recognise common difficulties in eating and drinking in the older person
- Initiate first-line dietary advice and food first interventions to improve nutritional status of the older person

S. Jones (✉)
Office of Teaching and Learning, Coventry University, Coventry, England
e-mail: stacey.jones@coventry.ac.uk

© Springer Nature Switzerland AG 2021
W. McSherry et al. (eds.), *Understanding Ageing for Nurses and Therapists*,
Perspectives in Nursing Management and Care for Older Adults,
https://doi.org/10.1007/978-3-030-40075-0_8

8.2   Introduction

Nutrition is important in supporting health and well-being across the lifespan, and a healthy balanced diet is advocated to optimise health, prevent disease and maintain a good nutritional status. However, what is considered a healthy balanced diet for the general population requires tailoring to meet the individual needs of different populations; this chapter will focus on nutritional recommendations for adults over 60 years old. See Fig. 8.1 that highlights the learning objectives.

As we age, nutritional requirements change due to complex biological processes that occur (see Chap. 2), as well as changes in health status. Older people may experience one or more of the following that may affect nutritional intake and negatively impact on their nutritional status:

- A reduction in thirst perception or reduced appetite due to changes in taste or food preferences [1]
- Early satiety, meaning they are unable to eat large amounts of food at one sitting
- Gastrointestinal problems such as nausea, bloating, gastric pain, malabsorption, constipation or oesophageal reflux
- Difficulties in eating including problems like chewing, possibly as a result of dental caries or ill-fitting dentures, degeneration of the oral mucosa and reduced saliva production, or swallowing difficulties, which may require texture-modified food and assessment by a speech and language therapist [1]
- Problems with dexterity, tremors, vision, strength or coordination, which may limit their ability to self-feed and may need assistant or adapted equipment [2]
- Memory or cognitive impairment may lead to food avoidance, food refusal or forgetting to eat and drink. This may also cause changes in food preferences,

Fig. 8.1 Learning objectives

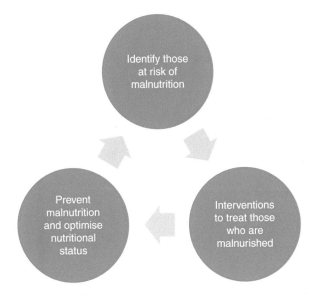

heightened anxiety around mealtimes and behavioural challenges such as hiding or throwing food or aggressive behaviour around mealtimes

- Physical impairment such as frailty or disability as well as social, mental health or physiological difficulties, which may adversely impact activities such as shopping for groceries, preparing food or cooking; requiring assistant from family or external agencies
- Emotional impact from social isolation, loneliness, boredom, depression or bereavement that may reduce motivation to eat, drink or general self-care [1]
- Poverty is common in the older population and may dictate what food is purchased and, therefore, restrict food choice and intake [2]
- Increased calorie requirements during acute illness, following trauma or in chronic disease

Therefore, small adaptations to mealtimes and food provision may enable people experiencing difficulties with eating and drinking to consume a diet that is able to meet their nutritional requirements and maximise their nutritional status.

If nutritional requirements are not met, individuals may experience weight loss, altered body composition and nutritional deficiencies, also known as malnutrition, which is associated with adverse effects on functional and clinical outcomes. Malnutrition in older people is often under-recognised because many people perceive low body weight and unplanned weight loss to be a normal part of ageing. Early identification of those at risk of malnutrition is recommended through the use of validated screening tools to prevent and treat malnutrition.

National Institute for Health and Care Excellence (NICE) (QS24 Nutritional Support in Adults (2012) states that all care services must take responsibility for the identification of people at risk of malnutrition and provide nutrition support for everyone with an indicated need. It is important that an integrated approach is taken across the multidisciplinary team to deliver high-quality care to adults who need nutrition support [3]. Good nutrition support services are crucial in patients at risk of malnutrition, and in many cases nutrition support services are provided as part of a wider care package to treat the underlying cause of malnutrition or manage the increased risk of malnutrition [4].

European Society for clinical nutrition and metabolism (ESPEN) guidelines on clinical nutrition and hydration in geriatrics, recommend all older persons should be routinely screened for malnutrition in order to identify risk early [2]. NICE guidelines [4] recommend screening for risks of malnutrition in all hospital inpatients on admission and all outpatients at their first clinic appointment. Screening should take place at GP visits to ensure early identification at every opportunity. Screening should be repeated weekly for inpatients and when there is clinical concern for outpatients. People in care homes should be screened on admission and repeated every 3 months or where there is clinical concern [2, 4]. The Mini Nutritional Assessment tool (Nestle Nutrition Institute) [5] and Malnutrition Universal Screening Tool [6] are commonly validated screening tools suitable for detecting those at risk of malnutrition.

A food first approach is recommended as a first-line intervention to correct nutritional deficiencies and maintain enjoyment of normal eating and drinking habits, whilst improving intake and preventing the adverse effects of malnutrition. Unnecessary dietary restrictions such as for diabetes or cholesterol lowering should generally be avoided as they may limit dietary intake and have been shown to be less effective with increasing age [2]. Liberalisation of diet prescriptions for older adults in the long-term may enhance nutritional status and quality of life [2].

8.3   Malnutrition

Malnutrition is defined as a deficiency or excess of nutrients such as energy, protein, vitamins and minerals, causing measurable adverse effects on body composition, function or clinical outcome, and is both a cause and a consequence of ill health [4]. Malnutrition in older adults is likely to relate to under-nutrition caused by compromised intake or assimilation of nutrients, in association with acute or chronic inflammation, leading to altered body composition and diminished biological function [7].

Unintentional weight loss is a common indicator of malnutrition in older adults, and significant weight loss is linked to reduced morbidity and mortality, particularly in those with a low BMI. There must be priority to obtain repeated weight measures over time to identify trajectories of decline, maintenance and improvement. It is important to recognise the pace of weight loss by determining the period of time the weight loss spans [7]. Percentage weight loss is calculated using the following equation:

$$\frac{\text{Original weight} - \text{current weight}}{\text{Original weight}} \times 100$$

However, changes in body weight do not always reflect changes in body composition; therefore, muscle mass is used as a measure to detect loss of fat-free mass. The decline in muscle mass is generally an indicator of reduced muscle function. Magnetic resonance imaging (MRI), computed tomography (CT) and dual-energy X-ray absorptiometry (DXA) are considered to be gold standards for non-invasive assessment of muscle quantity/mass, however, these tools are not commonly used in clinical practice due to high-equipment costs and lack of portability [8]. Bioelectrical impedance analysis (BIA) is considered a more user friendly and reliable tool to use in practice to measure fat-free mass. Physical examination or anthropometric measures of calf or mid-arm circumference require minimal specialist equipment or training and are good predictors of mortality. The cut-off points for diagnosis of malnutrition in older adults are <31 cm for calf circumference [8] and < 23.5 cm for mid-upper arm circumference [6].

There are several diagnostic criteria for diagnosing malnutrition including ESPEN guidelines (2015) [9] (*see* Box 8.1) and NICE [4] (*see* Box 8.2).

Box 8.1: ESPEN (2015) criteria for diagnosis of malnutrition; one of the following two criteria must be met:
1. BMI <18.5 kg/m^2
   OR
2. Unintentional weight loss >5% over 3 months or >10% over any period of time
   AND
   BMI <20 kg/m^2 (<70 years old) or <22 kg/m^2 (>70 years old)
   OR

Low fat-free mass index (FFMI) <15 kg/m^2 males and <17 kg/m^2 females

Box 8.2: NICE [4] criteria for diagnosis of malnutrition; any one of the following criteria must be met:
1. BMI <18.5 kg/m^2
   OR
2. Unintentional weight loss >10% within the last 3–6 months
   OR
3. BMI <20 kg/m^2 and unintentional weight loss >5% within the last 3–6 months

Until recently, there has been no single-existing approach or consensus that is commonly used for diagnosis globally. A working group; Global Leadership Initiative on Malnutrition (GLIM) was set up in 2016 to agree consensus on a definition and diagnostic criteria, which was published in 2019. The following diagnostic criteria were agreed upon [7] (*see* Box 8.3).

Box 8.3: GLIM criteria for the diagnosis of malnutrition: the individual must satisfy at least one criterion from the phenotype criteria and one criterion from the aetiologic criteria [7]
1. **Phenotype Criteria:**
   - Weight loss >5% with the past 6 months or >10% over 6 months
   OR
   - BMI <20 kg/m^2 (<70 years old) or <22 kg/m^2 (>70 years old)
   OR
   - Reduced muscle mass
2. **Aetiologic Criteria:**
   - Reduced food intake or assimilation: <50% of energy requirements for >1 week or any reduction for >2 weeks

OR
- Any chronic GI condition that adversely impacts food assimilation or absorption

OR
- Inflammation from acute disease/injury or chronic disease-related

Once malnutrition has been identified, first-line advice should be implemented to prevent further decline and promote optimisation of nutritional status. If required, a more comprehensive nutrition assessment should be carried out by an appropriately training professional such as a registered dietitian, which can provide the bases for an individualised nutritional care plan to be devised.

8.3.1   Causes of Malnutrition

Due to many factors, nutritional intake is often compromised in older persons and the risk of malnutrition increased. Anorexia of ageing, reduced dietary intake, impaired assimilation of nutrients combined with the effects of catabolic disease and inflammation can rapidly lead to malnutrition if untreated. Identifying the underlying causes of malnutrition can guide appropriate interventions to treat malnutrition.

Inflammation alters metabolism including elevation of resting energy expenditure and increased muscle catabolism leading to increased risk of malnutrition [7]. Acute inflammation such as from trauma, burns and major infections can be severe in nature. Indicators of inflammation may include fever, elevated energy expenditure and negative nitrogen balance. Chronic diseases such as congestive heart failure, COPD, obesity, rheumatoid arthritis, chronic kidney disease, liver disease or cancer are associated with mild-moderate inflammation over a prolonged period. Laboratory indicators of inflammation include serum C-reactive protein (CRP), albumin or pre-albumin [7].

Reduced dietary intake is common in older people, due to many factors including poor oral health, medication side effects, depression, dysphagia, gastrointestinal complaints, anorexia and inadequate nutrition support [7].

8.3.2   Prevalence of Malnutrition

There are estimated to be around 1.3 million people aged over 65 who are malnourished or at risk of malnutrition in the UK, and the vast majority (93%) of these live in the community; many of them unknown to healthcare services [10].

Analysis by the British Association of Parenteral and Enteral Nutrition (BAPEN) of data from nutrition screening from 2007 to 2011 shows that [11]:

- 25–34% of patients admitted to hospital are at risk of malnutrition.
- 30–42% of patients admitted to care homes are at risk of malnutrition.
- 18–20% of patients admitted to mental health units are at risk of malnutrition.

A report by BAPEN estimated annual public health and social care costs associated with malnutrition at £19.6 billion in England in 2011–2012, more than 15% of the total public expenditure on health and social care [10]. About half of this expenditure is on people >65 years [10]. Malnourished individuals were estimated to require healthcare expenditure 3.36 times greater than a person who was not malnourished [10].

8.3.3 Consequences of Malnutrition

Inadequate nutrition contributes to the progression of many diseases and is also regarded as one important contributing factor in the complex aetiology of sarcopenia and frailty [2]. Loss of muscle mass, strength and physical functioning leads to a reduced ability to perform basic activities of daily living, increases risk of falls and has adverse effects on quality of life and independence [2].

Consequences of malnutrition include increased susceptibility to infection, increased hospital admissions, greater length of hospital stay as well as increased likelihood of readmission to hospital [10]. Malnourished patients are at a higher risk of developing pressure ulcers and reduced recovery from illness [4].

8.4   Eating for Healthy Ageing and Preventing Malnutrition

Older people have similar nutritional needs as younger people for most micronutrients (vitamins and minerals), but their basal metabolic energy needs may be lower, while their protein needs may be higher, meaning that older people are likely to require a 'nutrient-dense' diet. Older people are at increased risk of micronutrient deficiencies due to an increasing prevalence of gastrointestinal diseases, accompanied by reduced nutrient bioavailability (e.g. atrophic gastritis, impaired vitamin B12, calcium and iron absorption); therefore, deficiencies should be corrected by supplementation [2].

In addition, older people may be unable to eat large amounts of food at one sitting. Therefore, more frequent and smaller meals including all essential nutrients may be appropriate. Eating alone and loneliness can also affect appetite, therefore, social eating should be encouraged wherever possible in an environment conducive to eating. Often in care settings, mealtimes are set, however, to maximise intake, there should be flexibility around individual preferences to timing and frequency of meals. Eating a nutrient-dense diet, together with regular exercise can help maintain body weight, muscle strength and independence.

Table 8.1 provides more detailed recommendations and guidance about nutrients. 'Eating for health' means a diet containing:

Table 8.1 Nutrients

Nutrient	Recommendations	Practical guidance
Energy	To maintain a healthy body weight, people need to consume enough calories each day to meet their total daily energy expenditure. In healthy individuals, this is estimated to be around 25–35 kcal/kg body weight per day [4]. However, this will depend upon physical activity levels, metabolic stress and disease and absorptive capacity and is likely to be higher in patients with chronic disease	Daily calorie intake can be increased by adding energy-dense food to a person's usual diet by adding foods that are high in fat (cream, cheese, butter, margarine, full-fat milk, oils. Avoid low-fat products)
Protein	Adults >65 years old have increased protein requirements, with a recommended intake of 1.2 g–1.5 g/kg/day [12]. Many older adults do not routinely consume enough protein to meet their nutritional needs. Insufficient protein intake can lead to a decline in muscle mass and strength leading to sarcopenia	Aim to serve a protein-rich food at each meal time. Protein-rich food include: Meat (or meat substitute), fish, beans, pulses, egg, dairy products (cheese, yogurt and milk), tofu, nuts and nut butters. Encourage regular milky drinks. Dried milk powder can be added to milky products, custard, sauces or drinks to further increase the protein content without increasing the volume. Oily fish are a good source of omega-3 fatty acids, which have anti-inflammatory properties and are good for heart health. Aim for at least 1–2 portions of oily fish per week. Oily fish include mackerel, salmon, trout, fresh tuna (not tinned), pilchards and sardines
Micro-nutrients	Aim for a balanced intake of vitamins and minerals. If there is concern about the patient consuming a balanced diet, a complete daily multivitamin and mineral supplement should be considered. Encourage 2–3 portions of dairy food each day to meet calcium requirements and keep bones strong and healthy. Vitamin D supplementation is recommended for all older people of 10 μg of vitamin D per day to maintain bone health [13]	Offer a small portion of vegetables alongside meals or incorporated into recipes. Offer fruit-based puddings, snacks or fruits as addition to breakfast cereal. Fruit and vegetables can be in the form of frozen, dried, tinned or fresh for convenience. Fruits and vegetables are low in calories, therefore, fortifying them with energy-dense food such as butter, olive oil, salad cream, mayonnaise (on vegetables and salad items) or honey, sugar, jam, peanut butter, cream, ice cream or custard (on fruit) will increase overall energy consumption

Table 8.1 (continued)

Nutrient	Recommendations	Practical guidance
Fluids	Older adults require 30 ml/kg/day [4] This is approximately 1.5–2.5 L (about 8 × 200 ml glasses) a day depending on climate and activity levels All fluids including fizzy drinks, milk, squash, tea and coffee and alcoholic beverages. All count towards fluid intake Dehydration is common in older people, especially those with dementia. Dehydration may lead to UTIs causing further delirium and increase risk of falls [14]	Ensure drinks are accessible throughout the day Try adding squash to water to enhance flavour Use adapted cups to improve dexterity. Clear containers may remind the patient to drink Encourage energy-dense fluids for those at risk of malnutrition Encourage fluid through food such as sauces, soups, fruits, jellies, yoghurts and ice cream

- Three to four meals with additional between meal snacks if needed
- At each meal:
  - Food rich in starchy carbohydrate and fibre
  - Food rich in high-quality protein
  - Fruits and vegetables
  - Food containing calcium and vitamin D (to support bone health)
- At least eight mugs/glasses (200 ml) of fluid throughout the day every day, which may mean drinking more fluid than some older people are used to

8.5 Nutritional Interventions to Treat Malnutrition

Oral nutrition can be supported by practical interventions, education, nutritional counselling, food modification and oral nutritional supplements [2]. Individualised approaches should be developed to allow optimised personal care focused on the patient's specific needs. Where possible, involving the patient in decision-making using appropriate communication tools to enable this [14].

It is important to aim to maintain a patient's ability to eat and drink as close to a normal diet for as long as possible to maximise the positive associations such as social, behavioural, comfort and enjoyment that is related to eating and drinking. A 'food first' approach is encouraged to increase the nutritional quality of the diet as well as encouraging additional intake [2]. Interventions to increase nutritional intake in patients with poor appetite are outlined in Table 8.2. The success and appropriateness of the intervention will be dependent on the individual patient and should be implemented alongside the recommendations of a qualified health professional following a detailed assessment of the individual's needs.

Table 8.2 Dietary interventions to prevent or treat malnutrition in older adults

Food first approaches
- Food fortification (adding nutrient dense foods to meals to increase nutrient content without significantly increasing volume - see table 8.1)
- Small frequent meals and snacks
- Finger foods that can be easily picked up without the use of cutlery (such as sandwiches, porkpie, cheese, crisps, nuts and dried fruit)
- Texture modification such as softer foods, blended, or adding sauces (if swallow difficulties are suspected, refer to a speech and language specialist)
- Strong flavours and smells, or sweeter food may be preferred [1]
- Avoid unnecessary dietary restrictions [16]

Behavioural/environmental interventions
- Encouragement talk
- Feeding assistance
- Colour-contrasting plates, tablecloths and place mats
- Adapted cutlery to support with dexterity
- Comfortable environment, pleasant mealtime experience, napkins, ceramic plates, not plastic trays
- Social eating with others
- Serve familiar and traditional food and smells
- Distraction-free
- Relaxing music [15]
- Involving the person in meal preparation or setting the table

Oral nutritional supplementation
- Oral nutritional supplement drinks—milk-based, juice-based, puddings- or yogurt-based, jelly-based, small volume, powders, sweet, savoury or flavourless to help meet nutritional requirements in patients who are unable to meet requirements through dietary manipulation. Only consider once all food first approaches have been implemented and evaluated [16]
- Oral nutritional supplements should provide a minimum of 400 kcal a day and 30 g protein and should be given for a minimum of 1 month [2]
- Consider daily multivitamin and mineral supplement for all adults who are not likely to be getting a full balanced diet [4]
- Provide Vitamin D supplementation 10 μg a day for all older adults [13] to support bone and muscle health

8.5.1 Food Fortification

For patients who are unable to meet their nutritional requirements through their current dietary intake, the aim is to fortify their intake or to increase the quality and density of nutrients. It is important to remember the aim is to maximise both energy density as well as nutrient density, therefore, continue to encourage a balanced diet.

8.5.2 Finger Food

Patients with dementia or those who are frail may experience problems with dexterity or hand eye coordination, therefore, may struggle to use cutlery to cut up food or transfer food to the mouth [2]. Serving food that can be easily picked up and eaten by hand may encourage the patient to consume food at meal and snack times. Food items such as sandwiches, fish fingers, sausages, pork pie, quiche, cheese cubes, vegetable sticks and dips, biscuits or sliced fruit may be appealing for patients with dexterity problems.

8.5.3 Enhanced Flavours and Smells

Ageing has a marked impact on appetite, weight loss and malnutrition due to complicated alterations in peripheral sensing and central processing. Older people have altered satiety signals, therefore, may have dampened appetite and poor appetite regulation in relation to calorie deficit [1].

Peripheral loss of taste/odour receptors or neurons causes significant deficits in the perception of taste preferences, quality, intensity and valence [1]. Patients with dementia have been found to have a strong preference for sweeter food and stronger flavours, which might be different to their pre-illness preferences [1].

8.5.4 Texture Modification

Modifying the textures of food in the diet can allow patients to continue to eat food that they enjoy and support them to meet their nutritional requirements. Soft food such as egg, fish, mashed potato, porridge or cereals soaked in milk, slow-cooked stews and food in sauces or even blended food may be preferred for people with problems chewing, possibly because of fatigue from prolonged mastication, mouth pain, dental caries or ill-fitted dentures.

Dysphagia is common, particularly in the later stages of dementia. Patients may have difficulties chewing food, moving food around the mouth to form a bolus or coordination of the swallow leading to aspiration. Patients may present with recurrent chest infections, refusing to eat, holding food in their mouth or food avoidance behaviours. Communication difficulties are prevalent in patients during the later stages of dementia, and it is important to remember that aspiration may occur without symptoms (i.e. silent aspiration). All patients with suspected dysphagia should be referred to a speech and language therapist for individualised advice on safe and appropriate texture modification in line with International Dysphagia Diet Standardisation Initiative (IDDSI) standards [14].

It is important to be aware that texture modification is associated with lower daily energy, protein and fluid intake, often due to food presentation being less appealing, reduced energy density and increased volumes of food needing to be consumed due to the addition of liquids; however, this can be mitigated with simple techniques. When blending food, keep individual foods separate to maintain individual flavours or use moulds to shape food to look like their original form to add visual appeal. Using energy-dense fluids such as full-fat milk or cream when blending will fortify meals and increase energy density.

8.6   Behavioural and Environmental Interventions

Environmental and behavioural modifications for increasing food and fluid intake in people with dementia include promotional activities around food intake, education of nurses, positive encouragement during mealtimes and self-feeding programmes, however, there is a lack of high-quality evidence in this area [17]. Protected mealtimes in hospitals to provide interruption-free mealtimes may enhance food intake, and assistance with mealtimes for those who require support has been shown be effective in increasing nutritional uptake [18]. Cooking from fresh and having the smells of the cooking may encourage food uptake in care homes, and food should be visually appealing.

Mealtime interventions in care homes focus on improving the mealtime routine, experience and environment for older adults. Interventions that have been shown to be effective include playing relaxing music, encouraging social eating, positive encouragement from staff at mealtimes and using verbal cues to prompt eating. As well as replicating a homely mealtime experience by using plates rather than trays, having napkins and tablecloths can enhance the mealtime experience and enjoyment. Changing the lighting, and increasing visual contrast with coloured plates and placemats can increase intake in those with visual impairments or with dementia. Offering more choice and autonomy to patients through serving food at the table, may encourage greater intake of food if people are empowered to choose their own food [1, 2].

8.6.1   Exercise and Preventing Sarcopenia

Sarcopenia is a progressive and generalised skeletal muscle disorder that is experienced through normal ageing, and is accelerated by physical inactivity or poor nutritional intake. It is associated with increased likelihood of adverse outcomes including falls, fractures, physical disability and mortality [8]. The European Working Group on Sarcopenia in Older People (EWGSOP) [8] recommend the use of the self-reporting SARC-F questionnaire as a screening tool to identify those at risk of sarcopenia. Responses are based on the patient's perception of their limitations in strength, walking ability, rising from a chair, stair climbing and experiences with falls.

A loss of muscle strength is used to diagnose sarcopenia. Low grip strength is a powerful predictor of poor patient outcomes and can be measured easily using a handheld dynamometer. Grip strength cut-off points for the diagnosis of sarcopenia are <27 kg men and <16 kg women [8].

The chair stand test (also called chair rise test) can be used as a proxy for leg strength. The chair stand test measures the amount of time needed for a patient to rise five times from a seated position without using his or her arms. Since the chair stand test requires both strength and endurance, this test is a qualified but convenient measure of strength. The cut-off point for diagnosis of sarcopenia is >15 s for five rises [8].

Reflective Questions

- Task 1—Think about recent patients that you have come into contact with who had lost weight and had poor nutritional intake. What actions did you take to address this?
- How did you try to understand the reason behind the patient's difficulties with eating and drinking? What would you do differently next time you come across a patient who has lost weight and has a poor nutritional intake?
- Task 2—Imagine a family member close to you has lost interest in eating and drinking, and you have noticed them losing weight gradually over the past 6 months. Despite encouraging them with food, they are still not able to increase their intake; you are now concerned with their frailty. How do you feel? What support might you expect from a healthcare professional? How could you be involved in the nutritional care plan?
- Task 3—How would you explain the importance of good nutrition and hydration to your patients and their families in order to motivate them? How would you ensure nutrition and hydration are included as a crucial part of the care plan for older patients? How can you promote better nutrition and hydration in your setting?

Combined interventions incorporating progressive resistance exercise (at least twice per week) and nutritional optimisation (particularly meeting protein requirements of 1.2–1.5 g/kg/day) have been shown to have positive outcomes on improving muscle mass, muscle strength and physical function [12, 19, 20].

8.7 Summary of Main Points

A holistic, multidisciplinary approach is needed to ensure high-quality nutritional care, and support is provided to all older people as an integral part of the care process. A detailed and thorough assessment of nutritional status as well as regular screening and monitoring of weight is vital to ensure the nutritional status of the patient can be optimised. Interventions should focus on a food first approach and consideration given to the social, environmental and psychological aspects of eating and drinking as well as the physiological factors affecting dietary intake. Interventions should be implemented immediately and monitored closely, and account for the natural ageing progression and changing needs of the individual. Referral to a dietitian is advised for those at high risk of malnutrition in line with local referral guidelines.

8.8 Suggested Reading

Further resources on providing first-line nutritional interventions for the prevention and treatment of malnutrition can be found on the following websites:

- British Association of Parenteral and Enteral Nutrition (BAPEN) website: https://www.bapen.org.uk/nutrition-support/nutrition-by-mouth
- Malnutrition pathway website: https://www.malnutritionpathway.co.uk/copd
- British Dietetics Association (BDA) food fact sheets: https://www.bda.uk.com/foodfacts/malnutrition

References

1. Nifli A (2018) Appetite, metabolism and hormonal regulation in normal ageing and dementia. Diseases 6(3):66
2. Volkert D, Beck AM, Cederholm T, Cruz-Jentoft A, Goisser S, Hooper L, Kiesswetter E, Maggio M, Raynaud-Simon A, Sieber C, Sobotka L, Asselt D, Wirth R, Bischoff S (2018) ESPEN guideline on clinical nutrition and hydration in geriatrics. Clin Nutr 38:10–47
3. NICE (2012) Nutrition support in adults [QS24]. https://www.nice.org.uk/guidance/qs24. Accessed 20 Sept 2019
4. NICE (2006) Nutrition support for adults: oral nutrition support, enteral tube feeding and parenteral nutrition [CG32]. https://www.nice.org.uk/Guidance/cg32. Accessed 20 Sept 2019
5. Nestle Nutrition Institute (NNI). Mini nutritional assessment tool. https://www.mna-elderly.com/. Accessed 23 Sept 2019
6. British Association of Parenteral and Enteral Nutrition (BAPEN) (2018) Malnutrition Universal Screening Tool (MUST). https://www.bapen.org.uk/screening-and-must/must/must-toolkit/the-must-itself. Accessed 23 Sept 2019
7. Cederholm T, Jensen GL, Correia M, Gonzalez M, Fukushima R, Higashiguchi T, Baptista G, Barazzoni R, Blaauw R, Coats A, Crivelli A, Evans D, Gramlich L, Fuchs-Tarlovsky V, Keller H, Llido L, Malone A, Mogensen KM, Morley JE, Muscaritolo M, Nyulasi I, Pirlich M, Pisprasert V, de van der Schueren MAE, Siltharm S, Singer P, Tappenden K, Velasco N, Waitzberg D, Yamwong P, Yu J, Van Gossum A, Compher C (2019) GLIM criteria for the diagnosis of malnutrition – a consensus report from the global clinical nutrition community. J Cachexia Sarcopenia Muscle 10:207–217
8. Cruz-Jentoft J, Bahat G, Bauer J, Boirie Y, Bruyere O, Cederholm T, Cooper C, Landi F, Rolland Y, Sayer A, Schneider S, Sieber C, Topinkova E, Vandewoude M, Visser M, Zamboni M, Bautmans I, Baeyens J, Cesari M, Cherubini A, Kanis J, Maggio M, Martin F, Michel J, Pitkala K, Refinster J, Rizzoli R, Sanchez-Rodriguez D, Schols J (2019) Sarcopenia: revised European consensus on definition and diagnosis. Age Ageing 48:16–31
9. Cederholm T, Bosaeus R, Barazzoni R, Bauer J, Van Gossum A, Klek S, Muscaritoli M, Nyulasi I, Ockenga J, Schneider SM, de van der Schueren M (2015) Diagnostic criteria for malnutrition – an ESPEN consensus statement. Clin Nutr 34:335–340
10. Elia M (2015) The cost of malnutrition in England and potential cost savings from nutritional interventions: a report on the cost of disease-related malnutrition in England and a budget impact analysis of implementing the NICE clinical guidelines/quality standard on nutritional support in adults. https://www.bapen.org.uk/pdfs/economic-report-full.pdf
11. Russell, Elia (2012) Nutrition screening survey in the UK and ROI in 2011. BAPEN. https://www.bapen.org.uk/pdfs/nsw/nsw-2011-report.pdf. Accessed 20 Sept 2019
12. Duetz N, Bauer J, Barazzoni R, Biolo G, Boirie Y, Bosy-Westphal A, Cederholm T, Cruz-Jentoft A, Krznaric Z, Nair S, Singer P, Teta D, Tipton K, Calder C (2014) Protein intake and exercise for optimal muscle function with aging: recommendations from the ESPEN Expert Group. Clin Nutr 33:929–936

13. Scientific Advisory Committee on Nutrition (SIGN) (2016) Vitamin D and health report. https://www.gov.uk/government/publications/sacn-vitamin-d-and-health-report. Accessed 20 Sept 2019

14. NICE (2018) Dementia: assessment, management and support for people living with dementia and their carers [NG97]. https://www.nice.org.uk/guidance/ng97. Accessed 20 Sept 2019

15. Whear R, Abbott R, Thompson-Coon J, Bethel A, Rogers M, Hemsley A, Stahl-Timmins W (2014) Effectiveness of mealtime interventions on behaviour symptoms of people with dementia living in care homes: a systematic review. J Post-Acute Long-Term Care Med 15(3):185–193

16. Volkert D, Chourdakis M, Faxen-Irving G, Fruhwald T, Landi F, Suominen M, Vandewoude M, Wirth R, Schneider S (2015) ESPEN guidelines on nutrition in dementia. Clin Nutr 34(6):1052–1073

17. Herke M, Fink A, Langer G, Wustmann T, Watzke S, Hanff AM, Burckhardt M (2018) Environmental and behavioural modifications for improving food and fluid intake in people with dementia. Cochrane Database Syst Rev (7):CD011542

18. Edwards D, Carrier J, Hopkinson J (2017) Assistance at mealtimes in hospital settings and rehabilitation units for patients (>65 years) from the perspective of patients, families and healthcare professionals: a mixed methods systematic review. Int J Nurs Stud 69:100–118

19. Cermak NM, Res PT, De Groot LCPGM, Saris WH, Van Loon LJC (2012) Protein supplementation augments the adaptive response of skeletal muscle to resistance-type exercise training: a meta-analysis. Am J Clin Nutr 96:1454–1464

20. Denison H, Cooper C, Sayer A, Robinson S (2015) Prevention and optimal management of sarcopenia: a review of combined exercise and nutrition interventions to improve muscle outcomes in older people. Clin Interv Aging 10:859

Continuity of Care

9

James Brockie and Carolyn Gair

Contents

9.1 Learning Objectives

This chapter will enable you to:

- Develop the reader's understanding of the benefits and challenges of inter-professional working between health and social care colleagues
- Increase the reader's knowledge of the roles and responsibilities of social workers and social care professionals in relation to hospital discharge and admission avoidance
- Enhance the reader's skills to work effectively with social workers and other social care professionals to promote the continuity of inpatient care

J. Brockie (✉) · C. Gair
Social Work, Staffordshire University, Stoke-on-Trent, England
e-mail: james.brockie@staffs.ac.uk; Carolyn.gair@staffs.ac.uk

© Springer Nature Switzerland AG 2021
W. McSherry et al. (eds.), *Understanding Ageing for Nurses and Therapists*,
Perspectives in Nursing Management and Care for Older Adults,
https://doi.org/10.1007/978-3-030-40075-0_9

9.2   Introduction to the Topic

The term 'Continuity of Care' refers to a continuous and consistent therapeutic relationship with a clinician or care manager, 'including providing and sharing information and care planning, and any coordination of care required by the patient' [1]. Whilst the term 'Continuity of Care' is predominantly used by health professionals, it is a concept which readily translates to social work. Research suggests that service users value having the same social worker involved in their care as it can support them to adjust to new environments [2] and transitions in their lives. There is also evidence that suggests that 'Relationship-Based Practice', which focuses on the relationship between a social worker and the service user that they are working with, rather than the procedural and administrative functions of the role, is effective when working with adults who are in need of care and support [3].

In the hospital setting, social workers play a central role in both admission avoidance and discharge. Like all professions, social work must be viewed through the lens of the social and historical context in which its practice is situated. Social work in England has its origins in what we would now understand to be the third sector, typically Christian charities providing support to people experiencing hardship. As the modern welfare state emerged after the Second World War, social workers found themselves in a pivotal role, supporting people to navigate the increasingly complex and bureaucratic welfare system and allocating scarce resources to those in the greatest need. Although social work is now a regulated profession, with its own evidence-base, and distinct set of professional values, social workers still retain a role as gatekeepers of services and funding. Whilst successive governments have explored the possibility of integrating health and social care, the two services remain separate and distinct. Further to this, the evidence that integrated working benefits patients/service users is limited [4] and actualising the organisational and cultural changes needed to truly integrate services can be problematic [5].

Although nurses, therapists, and social workers often work in partnership, there can be some ambiguity about the role of a social worker. This is unsurprising given that there are many definitions of what social work is, perhaps most widely recognised of which is the following:

> Social work is a practice-based profession and an academic discipline that promotes social change and development, social cohesion, and the empowerment and liberation of people. Principles of social justice, human rights, collective responsibility and respect for diversities are central to social work. Underpinned by theories of social work, social sciences, humanities, and indigenous knowledge, social work engages people and structures to address life challenges and enhance wellbeing. The above definition may be amplified at national and/or regional levels [6].

For many social workers, promoting people's rights and autonomy remains at the heart of good practice. Despite what many researchers have described as a shift towards managerial approaches to practice over recent decades, there has been a drive from within the profession to refocus on relationship-based practice [7]. In the UK, the government has produced a framework that reinforces this change of direction and identifies the fundamental knowledge and skills required of a social worker in adult services [8]. Subsequent policy documents reiterate the cultural shift that is required in health and social care organisations to ensure that care is person-centred [9]; however, Hollinrake [7] argues that the legal framework that underpins practice still adopts a neoliberal perspective and reinforces the role of the private sector in the provision of care and support of older people in England. For many researchers, the competitive nature of the free market and the profit motive of private companies are difficult to reconcile with the ambition of providing personalised care [10]. Further to this, the high turnover of staff in the sector can also contribute to the difficulties of providing continuity in the care that patients/service users receive [11]. It should also be recognised that there are differences in the way health and social care services are organised and delivered around the world.

Research by Tanner et al. [2] suggests that social work has moved from its traditional therapeutic roots involving long-term work with individuals and communities to a system of 'episodic case management'. In practice, cases are usually closed as soon as immediate risks are reduced or delayed, and there is limited scope to build lasting relationships with patients. Further to this, the evidence suggests that staff turnover and sickness is high in both the NHS and social care [12], which only serves to compound the problem. Finally, providing patients/service users with continuity in their care can be challenging to achieve because often staff work for different organisations. Furthermore, staff who work in hospitals do not necessarily provide services to patients when they are back at home. However, in some areas a new model of assessment, Discharge to Assess, has been implemented, where a patient's social care assessment is completed after discharge [13]. Again, there are regional and national variations in relation to how these assessments are undertaken.

With these limitations in mind, it may be worthwhile broadening our understanding of the concept of 'Continuity of Care', to extend from thinking of a patient having a single professional who manages their entire journey, to a team of staff who work collaboratively at different stages. In such a complex system involving different legislation, policy, and practices, all staff should communicate clearly and effectively with one another about their patients. In the fast-paced environment of a busy hospital, all staff must be mindful that their record keeping is factual, concise, and clearly presented, so that it can be understood by a range of different professionals. Further to this, the use of acronyms and medical jargons should be avoided.

Although practices vary between local areas, the role of a social worker in the UK might be best understood as follows: social workers operate under a legal framework, primarily the Care Act 2014 [14], and assess the care and support needs of adults whose independence and well-being may be compromised due to physical or mental impairments or safeguarding concerns. At a basic level, a social worker might become involved, where a patient may require care and support upon discharge, such as help with washing and dressing, meal preparation, managing their finances, or accessing the community. The role of the social worker is to establish whether a person has eligible needs for care and support through undertaking an assessment. They should then work with the patient, other professionals, and any other person that the patient would like to be involved to establish how best to meet the needs identified in the assessment.

In addition to assessing needs and coordinating patients' care and support, social workers lead enquiries into allegations of abuse [14]. This is rarely a straightforward process and can sometimes delay a patient's discharge. Sometimes, an episode of abuse can be the reason why a patient has ended up in hospital, for example, through neglect or a physical injury. It may be that a social worker will want the input of a health professional in their enquiry. A social worker may require the professional opinion of a nurse on a specific issue, they might also welcome a written assessment of a patient's health needs. A social worker might also value a nurse's input into a risk of assessment if the patient has complex medical conditions, which may increase the chances of them coming to harm outside of a hospital environment. This kind of inter-professional working is vital in safeguarding work. The government initiative *Making Safeguarding Personal* [15] stresses the importance of involving patients/service users in safeguarding enquiries. Research informs that it is important to establish what patients/service users want out of a safeguarding enquiry and to set goals with them, in order to increase resilience and reduce the number of repeat referrals [16].

9.3   Theory, Rationale, and Evidence Base

Research into the efficacy of social work interventions with adults in this context is patchy. At this juncture, it is worthwhile acknowledging that there is some debate about the nature of social work practice, specifically around whether social work is an art or a science. Most of the social work research is qualitative and small-scale. Indeed, some researchers reject the validity of 'scientific' research methods altogether. Hence, you will rarely encounter randomised control trials in social work research. A recent systematic review of the research on social work interventions in adult services found that there was a measurable benefit to patients from social work intervention in their care. Some of the reasons for this included a social worker's ability to provide education and counselling support to patients, as well as connecting them with community support [17]. This contributes to the continuity of care that patients receive.

The following section will explore those key skills and the evidence base for social workers in practice (Fig. 9.1):

9.3.1   Analysis

A core element of social work is in the analysis of information. Social workers must weigh up evidence that relates directly to the adult they are working with, as well as consider the social and environmental factors that are impacting on that person. For example, a social worker will need to meet with the person the assessment is considering but may also meet with anyone involved in their care (family/non-family members, nurses, occupational therapists) and consider wider ecological factors such as policies and benefit systems. A social worker will not just consider what is

Fig. 9.1 The social work
role in continuity of care

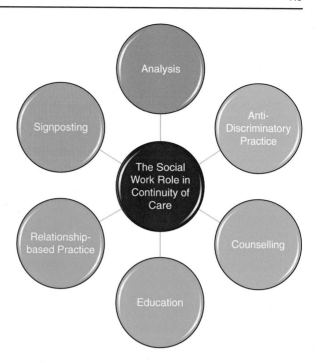

happening, but will also provide analysis around what this situation means for the person, how it impacts on them, and what then, is going to help meet this person's needs within the legal powers and duties of the social worker in that situation. Analysis also offers an opportunity to assess and manage risk, which is of paramount importance within safeguarding as well as regarding continuity of care. This involves reflection on (and synthesis of) the information gathered—information which often changes and evolves during an assessment. Social work assessments are often 'needs-led' in this way as the analysis focuses on that person and what they need. However, there may also be an element of research as the social worker must look at what is available in regard to services and which will best meet the needs of the person they are working with. Social workers must often also negotiate and advise depending on the resources available for that person, and this can be reflected within the analysis as well. This will all contribute positively to continuity of care for the person.

9.3.2 Anti-Discriminatory Practice

People experience discrimination for many reasons. It may be deliberate acts based in bigotry and intolerance, or it may unintentional, caused by ignorance to the ideological discriminatory discourses that exist within society. Thompson [18] reminds social workers that part of the social work task is to have and own an awareness of the discourses that exist and the layers of discrimination and oppression that ensues.

A person could live with multiple layers of discrimination and oppression, which will impact on them socially as well as emotionally, and this should be considered within a social worker's assessment and intervention when working around continuity of care. Being anti-discriminatory is a core value and responsibility in social work [18], and therefore, it is not enough to just not be discriminatory: social workers must stand up against it and challenge the cultural and structural systems that create and reinforce personal discrimination. At a personal level, this may include challenging the attitudes of others, advocating and fighting for access to services upon discharge from hospital, and educating the person around what services they are entitled to receive.

9.3.3 Counselling

Counselling is certainly not unique to the social work profession; however, counselling skills are crucial for all social workers, especially when working with adults experiencing crisis [3]. The theoretical frameworks that underpin social work practice inform social workers working with people across the lifespan. Although ageing can be a positive experience for some, it is also a time of grief and loss for some older people for a variety of reasons including the death of a partner, feelings of isolation, and loneliness. Further to this, some of the physical and biological effects of ageing, such as declining health, can also have a detrimental emotional impact. Social workers can utilise their counselling skills to support older people who experience emotional difficulties and to explore the social dimensions of ageing with each adult they are working with. Boyd and Bee [19] posit that Levinson's theory is useful in this context as it suggests that people go through seasons of stability and transition or instability at various stages of life. A good assessment and intervention can help enable growth and change at any stage or season including when in transition between hospital, home, or community-based settings. Indeed, by using therapeutic and counselling skills, social workers can gain an in-depth understanding of a person's lived experience, which in turn contributes to a holistic assessment and care plan. This can be of particular importance for those experiencing grief or isolation, where the process of assessment with a social worker using counselling skills may be therapeutic in itself.

9.3.4 Education

Social workers can also play an important role in educating patients. This often involves education around medical and social terms being used by professionals, but also around the policies and processes in place. As a value-based profession, the empowerment of individuals is integral to the function and purpose of social work [20]. By explaining structures and processes, this can empower people to make informed decisions and can provide emotional reassurance if someone is confused about their situation. One such example of empowerment through education could be sharing information around delayed transfers of care (DTOCs). If a person is well and able to leave the hospital, they should not be delayed in doing so because they are waiting for transfer—this can cause unnecessary confusion and distress and can also prevent the admission of those in need. However, completing a thorough holistic assessment and when needed, agreeing on a care package, can be time-consuming for those being assessed and for social workers completing them. Ultimately, local authorities can be fined in relation to DTOCs, which can lead to conflicting priorities. By sharing some of this information with patients/service users, it may enable them to understand an organisational perspective of the situation and the urgency of the assessment. The National Institute for Health and Care Excellence (NICE) guidelines [21] highlight the necessity for communication and information sharing between professionals and with service users, and it is this communication and information sharing that informs and empowers the adult receiving services.

9.3.5 Relationship-Based Practice

Relationship-based approaches to social work have experienced a renaissance in recent years, perhaps as a response to the neoliberal context that social work has been operating within, but also perhaps due to the increased evidence base for effectiveness in working holistically and effectively. The underpinning message here is that building and maintaining relationships with people can result in successful social work when working with people across the lifespan. Dimes [3, p. 61] suggests that social workers can use their skills as 'a catalyst for change' and cites the following as being vital tools for relationship-based social work practice with adults: professionalism, openness, honesty, anti-discrimination, and active listening. These tools can heavily influence the quality of the interactions between social workers and the people that they work with. If people work with honesty and openness, actively listening with a professional ear, then a relationship can develop that will enable a thorough and person-centred assessment of need and risk. This extends to the inter-professional working that is so important to social work with adults, as well the relationship-based interactions with the adults receiving services. Conversely, evidence from serious case reviews and failures to safeguard individuals suggests that a breakdown in communication can lead to poor care and serious failures in hospitals [22, pp. 147–185]. Relationship-based practice now forms part of social work education and can be found in practice settings across social work organisations.

9.4 Signposting

It can often be pertinent for social workers to signpost people to using or making appointments with other services to ensure continuity of care. Under the Care Act 2014, a person must be 'eligible' for care and support, and it may be the case that they are eligible in relation to some of their needs but not all of them. In these instances, a social worker will research the most relevant and accessible service and direct the person to access that service. Furthermore, the key principles of the Care Act 2014 are to prevent, reduce, and delay the requirements for care, and therefore, a social worker may refer or signpost someone to a service that may prevent or reduce their need for services. This could include making a referral to a health professional or perhaps making use of the third sector or community-based group. An example of this in practice might be when a person has a specific need around smoking cessation and requests some support in this area. A social worker would refer or signpost the person to their GP or nurse specialist to meet this need. Or if a person was feeling isolated, it may be relevant to signpost to a community-led lunch club, for example, whilst assessing other care and support needs.

Practice Examples
Mrs. Jones

Mrs Jones is 89 years old and lives alone in a small flat in a small town in England. Mrs Jones is estranged from her son, who is her only living relative. They have not had contact for over 10 years. Mrs Jones has been in and out of hospital on a regular basis for the past 6 months. Mrs Jones tends to be admitted late at night in a confused state, usually after pressing her emergency alarm. One of the reasons for Mrs Jones' admissions has been urinary tract infections, but on most occasions, there is no medical reason for her to be in hospital. The last recorded medical notes state that Mrs Jones has 'dementia-like' symptoms, but she has no formal diagnosis. Further to this, the nurse in charge of the ward has recorded on several occasions that Mrs Jones is 'lonely and frightened at home alone'. The nurse has also documented that Mrs Jones is 'alert and well' whenever she wakes up in hospital.

In this case, the health and social care professionals involved in Mrs Jones's care need to work in partnership with her to resolve this situation. In England, the Mental Capacity Act 2005 requires everyone working with Mrs Jones to assume that she can make her own choices unless there is evidence that she is unable to make specific decisions for herself, irrespective of any diagnosis of dementia. This extends to all decisions, but in this case, we would focus on decisions around her care and treatment. Mrs Jones should be involved in all discussions about her needs and in developing a person-centred plan to support her to be discharged in a safe and effective fashion. In some local areas, there are health and social care staff who work collaboratively on 'admission avoidance' with patients who are at high risk of readmission. Not only does this kind or work promote interdisciplinary learning, but it is in the interests of the whole health and social care system that people are provided with support that meets their needs, in order to reduce the burden on hospital services. The key to success is working together and ensuring that all sources of support, whether these are funded by the NHS, the local authority, or through voluntary services, are thoroughly explored. It is also worthwhile gaining patients' consent to share any plans with those who may work with them in the community, for example, their GP, community nurses, mental health services, or social workers. This can help ensure that there is continuity in the care that patients receive.

Robert

Robert is a 66-year-old gentleman who has been in hospital after experiencing a stroke. Robert lives with his partner Brian in a large four-bedroomed property in the suburbs of a large city in England. Robert has made a very good recovery so far, although he struggles to speak clearly at times, and he needs some support when mobilising. With his consent, the nurse in charge has made a referral to the local authority for an assessment of Robert's needs. The Care Act 2014 places a duty on each local authority to undertake a holistic assessment of any adult with the appearance of a need for care and support. Inderjit, a social worker from the hospital assessment team, arranges to meet Robert, Brian, and the nurse in charge on the ward to begin an assessment of his needs. The assessment covers all areas of Robert's life, not just his health, but also his needs in relation to emotional well-being, his spiritual needs, relationships, finances, and social life, in addition to anything else that is important to Robert. It is vital that Inderjit's assessment is informed not only by Robert's view of his own needs, but also any assessments completed by the doctors, nurses, and therapists who have been working with him whilst he has been in hospital. Although some professionals worry about sharing information, most hospitals will have information-sharing agreements whereby they can share information about patients with social workers. In Robert's case, he is likely to have ongoing support from a speech and language therapist and a physiotherapist when he is discharged. Any care plans and therapy goals will need to be shared with Inderjit so that Brian and/or domiciliary care staff can be trained to support Robert to complete any exercises necessary to aid his recovery when he is back at home. Inderjit will also want to consider Brian's views and would offer him the opportunity to have a carer's assessment in his own right. In England, the Care Act 2014 gives service users the right to request the amount of money that it would cost to meet their care needs (their personal budget) paid to them as a direct payment, which they can spend on services to meet their care and support needs. Inderjit would talk to Robert about this and offer him support to manage his budget. Inderjit would also talk openly to Robert about how he wants his care needs to be met and by whom. Any care that is arranged for him at home should be personalised and consider his social and emotional needs, alongside practical day-to-day considerations.

Reflective Exercises
- Nurses and other health professionals often take a medical perspective on the needs of their patients. In the case of Mrs. Jones, consider the social and environmental challenges that have led to her hospital admission. What do you think could be done to help address some of these challenges?
- Robert and Brian are a same-sex couple and are likely to have experienced discrimination in their lives because of their sexuality. Consider the ethical duties upon you as a professional, how could you promote their rights and avoid discriminating against them?
- In this chapter, we have referred to some of the challenges that health and social care staff experience when they work inter-professionally. Consider the knowledge, skills, and values you will need to work collaboratively with Inderjit to achieve the best possible outcomes for Robert and Brian.

9.5 Taking It Further

1. What other factors would you need to consider if Robert was from a culture that did not usually accept domiciliary care from paid carers?
2. Consider the knowledge, skills, and values that you might need if Robert's stroke had affected him more significantly and he could no longer communicate verbally. How might the way that you work with him change?
3. You have already considered the knowledge, skills, and values you need to work collaboratively with a social worker. In the case of Mrs. Jones, what knowledge, skills, and values do you think Inderjit would need to work with you?

9.6 Summary

The value base of social work is well aligned to the caring values of the health professions, and this common ground can provide an opportunity for successful inter-professional working. This chapter has explored the concept of continuity of care from a social work perspective. The importance of inter-professional working in hospital discharge and transition to community-based care is well documented, and it is hoped that by sharing knowledge around the roles and responsibilities of social workers, this will enhance skills in working effectively to promote continuity of care and collaboration to achieve the best outcomes for patients/service users.

9.7 Suggested Further Reading and URLs

Age UK
 A national charity that works to improve the lives of older people and their carers. Their website includes useful fact sheets, research, and videos. [https://www.ageuk.org.uk/]

Aveyard H, Sharp, P. *A beginner's guide to evidence-based practice in health and social care*. 2nd. Maidenhead: Open University Press; 2013.

A useful guide to using evidence in practice for both health and social care professionals.

Cooper A, White E. (2017) *Safeguarding adults under the Care Act 2014*. London: Jessica Kingsley Publishers Ltd.; 2017.

A concise and accessible guide to adult safeguarding legislation, policy, and practice.

Feldon P. *The social worker's guide to the Care Act 2014*. St Albans: Critical Publishing Ltd.; 2017.

An accessible and informative text, aimed at social workers, but useful to anyone interested in the legal framework upon which care and support are provided to service users in England.

Holder, H. Managing the hospital and Social Care interface: interventions targeting older adults. www.newhealthfoundation.org/web/wp-content/uploads/2018/04/hospital-and-social-care-interface-final-web.pdf *(accessed 28 October 2019)*.

A useful report which evaluates different models of hospital discharge and makes recommendations for future practice.

Offord N, Harriman P, & Downes T. Discharge to assess: transforming the discharge process of frail older patients. *Future Healthcare Journal 2017*, 4 (1)

An informative journal article which explores the 'Discharge to Assess' model, which involves patients being discharged from hospital with a care package and then receiving their social work assessment at home.

Social Care Institute for Excellence

A range of freely accessible resources including practice guides, briefings, reports, and research summaries. Includes resources on personalisation, adult social work, and safeguarding. [https://www.scie.org.uk/]

Think Local, Act Personal

Website of the TLAP partnership. The site includes a number of resources (publications, videos, blogs) related to the personalisation of adult social care. [https://www.thinklocalactpersonal.org.uk/]

References

1. Freeman G, Hughes J. Continuity of care and the patient experience. https://www.kingsfund.org.uk/sites/default/files/field/field_document/continuity-care-patient-experience-gp-inquiry-research-paper-mar11.pdf. Accessed 28 Oct 2019
2. Taner D, Glasby J, McIver S (2015) Understanding and improving older people's experiences of service transitions: implications for social work. Br J Soc Work 45(7):2056
3. Dimes M (2019) Relationship-based social work with older people. In: Dix H, Hollinrake S, Meade J (eds) Relationship-based social work with adults. Critical Publishing, St. Albans, pp 59–76
4. Cameron A, Lart R, Bostock L, Coomer C (2014) Factors that promote and hinder joint and integrated working between health and social care services: a review of research literature. Health Soc Care Community 22(3):225–233
5. Phillipowsky DJ (2018) The perceptions regarding social workers from within an integrated trust in an age of austerity. J Integr Care 26(1):38–53

6. International Federation of Social Work. Global definition of social work. https://www.ifsw. org/what-is-social-work/global-definition-of-social-work/. Accessed 28 Oct 2019
7. Hollinrake S (2019) The legislative and policy context. In: Dix H, Hollinrake S, Meade J (eds) Relationship-based social work with adults. Critical Publishing, St. Albans, pp 26–46
8. Department of Health. Knowledge and skills statement for social workers in adult services. https://assets.publishing.service.gov.uk/government/uploads/system/uploads/attachment_ data/file/411957/KSS.pdf. Accessed 28 Oct 2019
9. Department of Health and Social Care. Adult social care: quality matters overview. https:// www.gov.uk/government/publications/adult-social-care-quality-matters-overview. Accessed 28 Oct 2019
10. Henderson F, Whittam G, Moyes D, Reilly C (2018) From charity to social enterprise: the marketization of social care. Int J Entrepreneur Behav Res 24(3):651–666
11. Skills for Care. The state of the adult social care sector and workforce in England. https://www. skillsforcare.org.uk/adult-social-care-workforce-data/Workforce-intelligence/publications/ national-information/The-state-of-the-adult-social-care-sector-and-workforce-in-England. aspx. Accessed 28 Oct 2019
12. Ravalier JM (2018) Psycho-social working conditions and stress in UK social workers. Br J Soc Work 49(2):371
13. Vernon M. NHS England's quick guide: discharge to assess and benefits for older, vulnerable people. http://www.nhs.uk/NHSEngland/keogh-review/Documents/quick-guides/Quick-Guide-discharge-to-access.pdf. Accessed 9 March 2020
14. Care Act 2014. http://www.legislation.gov.uk/ukpga/2014/23/contents/enacted. Accessed 9 March 2020
15. Local Government Association. Making safeguarding personal. https://www.local.gov.uk/our-support/our-improvement-offer/care-and-health-improvement/making-safeguarding-personal. Accessed 28 Oct 2019
16. Pike L (2016) Involving people in safeguarding adults. Totnes, Research in Practice for Adults
17. Moriarty J, Manthorpe J (2016) The effectiveness of social work with adults: a systematic scoping review. Kings College London, London
18. Thompson N (2016) Anti-discriminatory practice: equality, diversity and social justice, 6th edn. Palgrave, Basingstoke
19. Boyd D, Bee H (2015) Lifespan development, 7th edn. Pearson, Boston
20. British Association of Social Workers. Code of ethics. https://www.basw.co.uk/about-basw/ code-ethics. Accessed 20 March 2020
21. National Institute for Health and Care Excellence. Transition between inpatient hospital settings and community or care home settings for adults with social care needs. https://www. nice.org.uk/guidance/ng27/chapter/Recommendations#overarching-principles-of-care-and-support-during-transition. Accessed 28 Oct 2019
22. Mandelstam M (2013) Safeguarding adults and the law, 6th edn. Jessica Kingsley Publishers, London

Palliative and End of Life Care

10

Sarah H. Kagan

Contents

10.1   Learning objectives

This chapter will enable you to:

- Reflect on the nature of palliative and end of life care for older people.
- Identify resources to improve your capacity to provide palliative and end of life care to older people.
- Identify ways in which you can engage with older people to provide them palliative and end of life care that meets their needs and preferences.

S. H. Kagan (✉)
School of Nursing, Department of Biobehavioral Health Science, University of Pennsylvania, Philadelphia, PA, USA
e-mail: skagan@nursing.upenn.edu

© Springer Nature Switzerland AG 2021
W. McSherry et al. (eds.), *Understanding Ageing for Nurses and Therapists*,
Perspectives in Nursing Management and Care for Older Adults,
https://doi.org/10.1007/978-3-030-40075-0_10

10.2 Introduction

Palliative and end of life care for older people is among the most discussed health and social care topics in our ageing world. Popular media represent shifting preferences and changing understandings along with concerns about access to settings and resources for care. Scholars around the world, especially those from high income nations, aim to study and expose the full range of palliative and end of life care, from physiology of death and optimal clinical processes through experiences of elders receiving care, the bereaved, as well as clinicians and volunteers providing care. Rapidly evolving lay and professional literature challenge nurses and therapists who aim to develop their practice caring for older people in this domain. The sheer volume of original primary research and evidence syntheses may overwhelm clinicians seeking scientific currency, aiming to ensure evidence-based practice in palliative and end of life care.

Approaching development of one's own practice and contributing to a strong culture of practice within any health or social care setting requires a clear approach to define and improve palliative and end of life care. Considering factors that debunk myths, dispel ageism, clarify relationships, and employ best practices helps frame palliative and end of life care. Employing evidence in practice is commonly limited by scant, inapplicable, or poor-quality science. Often science is highly biomedical, risking depersonalisation and fragmentation of care. Nurses and therapists are typically well placed in health and social care systems around the world to identify and balance medicalisation of palliative and end of life care. These clinicians offer essential advocacy for older people who desire less medicalism, more holistic palliation, and more control over the place where and the nature of how, they close their lives. Nurses and therapists afford concrete, individual paths that humanise and personalise palliative and end of life care. Your actions as an individual nurse or therapist, taken with one older person at a time, collectively form a powerful contribution to palliative and end of life care—and indeed to health and social care more broadly—at the societal level.

This chapter addresses palliative and end of life care for older people with an overarching aim of dispelling ageism and offering fresh perspective for nurses and therapists seeking to develop their practice in this domain. The chapter begins with an overview of relevant theory and evidence for palliative and end of life care. This overview includes definitions, concepts, and controversies within palliative and end of life care, focusing on literature representing perspectives relevant around the world. A case study, drawing on essays written by Ruth McCorkle—a famed American cancer nurse scientist who lived and died with breast cancer—writing about her experiences and reflections, illuminates key concepts through a story where life and work intertwined. A practice example of palliative and end of life care at home, synthesises the theory and evidence discussed. A set of reflective exercises enable you to explore concepts presented for yourselves as people and as clinicians. Finally, ideas to take learning further provide you options to explore professional literature and your own communities to gain greater scholarly and practical knowledge of palliative and end of life care. Key terms are identified in **bold text** for ease in reading. Select terms are linked to readings for further study. Practical maxims for guiding palliative and end of life care are offered within the chapter in *italics*. Use these maxims—or principles—as <u>tips to improve your own practice</u>.

10.3 Theory and Evidence

Individuals, families, communities, and societies around the world understand palliative and end of life care in varying ways. Like birth, death is fundamentally human—a universal experience for us all. Similarly, death is profoundly personal. Each person's death is unique to the individual, a closing note to their life. In parallel, birth and death are fundamentally human and personal experiences utterly changed by medicalisation [1]. **Medicalisation** of death shapes palliative and end of life care as well as the social construction of end of life and death within any society. **Medicalisation** transforms natural processes in human life, altering expectations and confining these experiences to institutionalised settings where instrumental actions confound a simple desire for comfort and support. Death is now peculiarly a medical event, especially in high income and some low- and middle-income countries (LMICs) where allopathic Western healthcare dominates. Critically, many people may espouse preferences, as they age, for a death that conflicts with medicalised interpretation. Nonetheless, questions about desires for death at home, as realistic, arise as societies age demographically. Longevity often leaves many more people living alone, making that setting for palliative and end of life care logistically challenging [2].

End of life and death are constructed within specific societal and cultural contexts. Thus, resultant social constructions of end of life and death are specific to the place where and communities for which nurses and therapists provide care. Similarly, older people who are at the end of their lives share in and are informed by such social constructions as they face their own deaths. The anthropological concept of **social death** grounds illuminates the power of **social construction**. Social death sits in relation to biological death, occurring with, before, or after biological death. The relationship depends on social, cultural, familial, and individual precepts pertinent in an individual's death. For example, in cultures where religious traditions dictate that the biologically dead person is on display for some period, social death may not occur for days after biological death until burial or cremation occurs. Conversely, in other socio-cultural contexts, an older person living with a condition such as dementia may reach a point of social death long before biological death, calling to mind contemporary enquiries into concerns about dehumanising long-term institutional care in societies like Australia and the United Kingdom [3]. Medicalisation may mediate dissonance between biological and social death in both treatment and institutionalisation.

The contribution of medicalisation to the social construction of death makes defining palliative and end of life care essential to developing practice and improving care for older people as they close their lives. For the purposes of this chapter, **palliative care** is defined in this way. Palliative care focuses managing symptoms experienced by older people, aiding them in understanding their health and wellbeing, and supporting them emotionally, spiritually, and socially through professional and paraprofessional relationships, resources, and services. In this sense, **palliative care** requires knowledge of and relationship to the person. Conversely, **palliative care** defined in this manner does not require the services of a dedicated physician collaborator to occur. Similarly, this form of palliative care may occur outside of formal healthcare settings and palliative care programmes in, for example, social care and community-based programmes where therapists care for older people and provide support to their families. This definition implicitly reflects a current tension in the palliative care community about whether palliative care is in fact palliative medicine. The rise of palliative medicine arguably aligns with medicalisation of death. As such, it largely excludes or limits control for the older person while constraining contributions from nurses and therapists.

Importantly, the definition of palliative care used here rejects common attachment to diagnosis of serious or life-limiting illness with a short prognosis as defining eligibility for services. Attaching medical diagnoses and prognoses often conflicts with acknowledging proximate mortality inherent in later life. Such attachment diminishes the agency of the older person in defining their own life's end. Further, proscribing who is eligible for **palliative care** through restrictive diagnostic and prognostic criteria, then hampers access to palliative care for multimorbid elders whose medical problem list may belie overwhelming symptom burden and a foreshortened life span. Finally, defining palliative care in medical terms defies the essence of such care. Palliation means to relieve, lessen, or limit without curing or fixing the underlying problem. Nurses and therapists palliate symptoms, reactions, experiences, and meaning with and for people of all ages. **Palliative care** is arguably a tradition and character of care provided by nurses, therapists, social workers, chaplains, and other professionals. The tradition existed long before medicine staked its claim. Medical contributions to **palliative care** are certainly important. Nonetheless, the heart of such care is both human and personal; thus, practice of it sits with nurses, therapists and others.

Palliative rehabilitation is among the elements of palliative care least well characterised but frequently artfully practised. Societies with universal access to palliative and end of life care, and services where hospice philosophically guides end of life care, may offer more robust palliative rehabilitation than those where access is limited, and where hospice is simply a setting for care. For instance, scientific literature and clinical discourse on palliative rehabilitation appears stronger in the United Kingdom than in the United States. Fundamentally, both as a philosophical stance and an approach to care, palliative rehabilitation offers promising means to aid individuals to *live as well as they can for as long as they can* [4]. Nurses and therapists effectively collaborate in providing palliative rehabilitation for the older person. Rehabilitation is then central to **palliative and end of life care**, supporting the death the older person prefers.

10.3.1 End of Life and Palliative Care for Older People

In this chapter, **end of life** and **palliative care** are used largely synonymously. Older people live with a proximate mortality, whether they choose to acknowledge their own mortality and its relative but unspecified proximity. As a result, while **end of life** is most practically applied to the last days and hours of life where physiological change suggests that death is near, care up to and including those hours is both **palliative** and **end of life**. **End of life care** is then an extension of palliative care, temporally defined. However, some elements of **palliative care** at **end of life** are peculiar to those hours and intimately related to the person *dying as they lived*. Those elements include identifying and interpreting the **physiological indications of impending death** for the older person whose state of awareness is shifting rapidly, for loved ones who are often anxious, and for others attending at the **end of life**.

Connecting palliative and end of life care through proximate mortality obviates some **ageism** inherent in popular conceptions aiming to separate and constrict palliative and end of life care with medical diagnosis and prognosis. Gullette's moving personal account and analysis of ageism in healthcare reflects a larger literature substantiating institutional and individual ageism in various forms throughout health and social care [5]. Critically, **ageism** anchors—often invisibly—both under- and over-treatment of older people, subjecting them to incomplete access, delays, and diversions in care. **Ageism** creates iatrogenesis that prolongs discomfort from pain and other symptoms and risks premature death. **Ageism** in palliative and end of life care encompasses beliefs, attitudes, and actions taken by all actors involved in a situation, including nurses and therapists. **Ageism** directed toward older people as they anticipate and experience the close of their lives is frequently ambivalent and positively intended rather than being harsh and abusive [6]. For example, many people—professionals and lay people alike—feel protective toward an older person and frequently aim to protect that person from information and events they believe might be distressing. Kindly intended characterisations such as 'sweet' or 'cute' are generally ageist as well. Ambivalent, protective, and kind actions are, when based in perceptions of chronological age or frailty, nonetheless discriminatory. Reflective practices help identify personal, professional, and institutional ageism at hand in palliative and end of life care and develop plans to replace ageism with factual, non-discriminatory understandings and actions. Asking yourself *'would I think, feel, or act toward this person if they were 40 years younger?'* is a good place to begin reflecting in practice.

Like ageism, **moral judgement** is widely expressed and largely accepted or even embraced within end of life care as an appraisal of the quality of a death. The emergence of the **good death**, sometimes set in opposition to 'bad death', permeates palliative and end of life care clinical and social science literatures. In their important integrative review, Cottrell and Duggleby conclude that the notion of the **good death**, promulgated in science and care, constrains options for making death that for which the person hope [7]. While many laud the good death as guiding development of care at end of life, application of it deflects focus on the person with their hopes and fears about their death, substituting a mythical ideal. Usefully, asking about a **good death** may leverage a productive conversation with the older person about what they think is a good death. *The only good death for any individual is the death that avoids their fears and fulfils their hopes to the greatest extent possible.*

Person-centredness and **person-centred** care emerge logically from discussions of the human, the personal, and the social in palliative and end of life care. Fundamentally, however, person-centred is defined and applied in elastic ways, with varied implicit and explicit philosophical antecedents present [8]. Consequently, this chapter avoids particularistic interpretations of **person-centred** care and thus entanglement in various dialectics. Here instead, the person as individual and human being is wholly central to the who, why, and how of palliative and end of life care. The person defines themselves in identity, life, and relationships. They continue that self-definition, even with potential impingement on communication that may be life-long or a result of diseases and conditions with which they are living (e.g. dysarthria after oral cancer treatment or limited short-term memory in dementia) in palliative and end of life care. Principles, knowledge, and skills in communication are integral to education and socialisation of nurses and therapists. Capitalising on that education and socialisation, while drawing on expert colleagues such as occupational therapists and speech-language therapists, is essential to effective palliative and end of life care. Thinking and asking about the person and how they lived operationalises **person-centred** care by enabling nurses and therapists to better know the person in the manner they lived. Ask the person *'tell me about yourself and how you've lived your life'*. Ask those who knew them in the past and know them in the present who they are and how have they lived. Everything learned helps realise care, led by the maxim that *people die the way they lived* when given the opportunity.

10.3.2 Beyond Biomedical Evidence

Scientific evidence in palliative and end of life care abounds. **Evidence syntheses** emerge across a range of journals each month. However, the state of the science in specific phenomena such as transitions from curative treatment to end of life care, as well as more broadly across diagnostic populations, settings, and societies, offers scant bases for evidence-based practice in palliative and end of life care. Most evidence syntheses highlight conclusions about limited quality and quantity of evidence along with needs for more research. Most current **evidence syntheses in palliative and in end of life care** call into question the nature and aim of science in palliative and end of life care. The growing subspecialist emphasis on palliative and end of life care perhaps arises from profound medicalisation in these domains. Nurses and therapists may take a different view, situating themselves in the nursing metaparadigm and rehabilitative paradigm, respectively. Relying on their own paradigms enables nurses and therapists in making use of best practices and evidence drawn from beyond biomedical evidence to support therapeutic relationships, person-centredness, and palliation with and for older people. Reliance on the nursing metaparadigm and the rehabilitation paradigm also counterbalances allopathic emphasis on human health as an objective, singular state where a problem list codifies decrements to health. Within nursing and rehabilitation paradigms, **salutogenesis**, or health promotion, offers possibilities for health and wellbeing at the end of life. Here, palliative care need not address a problem list alone, settling for palliating the 'unfixable' person. Rather, relationships arise as central to health and wellbeing, underscoring growing evidence suggesting social connections are fundamental to long lives and highlighting health found through a sense of purpose and meaning in daily life. Nurses and therapists easily leverage therapeutic relationships to promote health and wellbeing and ably do so in later life. Focusing on advantages and strengths possessed by the older person situated in the life they are living and, at the end of which, they die still possessing facilitates palliative and end of life care. Seeing strength and highlighting advantages individualises palliative and end of life care. *An advantage inventory balances the medical problem list* in planning palliative and end of life care [9].

Case Study

End of life and the reality of death, as with birth, quickly reels beyond intellectual grasp when contemplated in human terms. So fundamental and elemental is death that it expands to touch almost all aspects of human existence. Reflection on death of an individual often provides insights by scaling the enormousness of end of life to personal terms. As we ourselves age as people, we are also nurses or therapists. Simultaneously, we hold many other important roles in daily life, roles that shape and reshape our identities. We often stand witness to those we know closing their lives in many different sorts of deaths. Reflecting on those experiences is crucial to developing our palliative and end of life care and to ourselves as people beyond our professional roles. Often reflecting together on the end of life and death of an individual is helpful in practice development. Collective reading among colleagues of classic memoirs like May Sarton's After the Stroke: A Journal [10] and newer works such as Raynor Winn's The Salt Path [11] offer rich possibility for shared reflection.

Ruth McCorkle, a famed American cancer nurse scientist, offers a remarkable case study through her life and her work, captured in her writings. In summer 2019, McCorkle died at the age of 79. She lived with breast cancer for decades and ultimately died of complications of the disease. McCorkle travelled to London in the 1970s and studied with Dame Cicely Saunders at St. Christopher's Hospice. McCorkle, as a nurse who first understood a diagnosis of cancer as a terminal condition—an expression little used in palliative care today—pondered death from a very early point in her scholarship. She wrote about an holistic approach to terminal illness with her mentor Jeanne Quint Benoliel in 1978, going on to write about the good death just a few years later [12, 13]. McCorkle enjoyed a stellar career in cancer nursing science, enjoying national and international acclaim in an era predating today's

24-h news media cycle. As cancer advanced later in McCorkle's life, she wrote an unplanned series of essays for the journal *Cancer Nursing* in which she proffered unselfconscious, particularistic, and incredibly illuminating insights. She lived with the effects of her cancer and repeated treatment. For example, she wore a lymphedema sleeve for many decades, partly a testament to the era in which she was treated, but never wrote about that experience. McCorkle wrote instead about close relationships with her nurses and others who cared for her while she maintained her identity as a nurse. Her insights culminate in a last essay (to be published posthumously) where she anticipates her own good death—a death very much on her own terms—by sharing a very intimate moment in which she dreams of her youngest son and her own father visiting her in her bedroom [14]. Colleagues who attended the memorial service held for McCorkle at Yale University School of Nursing reported she was unresponsive to those around her for only a very short time before she died. Known for her strong personality and definitive approach to life, McCorkle seemed to die as she lived. Her essays create a case study of intertwined social roles, clear identity, the journey of ageing with a serious diagnosis, anticipation and reflection on death, and the story of her own good death. McCorkle lucidly illustrates application of several key principles anchoring palliative and end of life care in her more recent essays.[1]

Practice Example

In a geriatric clinic, you meet Miss Mae Byrd, a woman in her tenth decade of life, and her younger sister Miss Louise who works part-time as a care assistant in a local nursing home. Miss Mae, as she prefers you to call her, is being treated with palliative radiotherapy for a secondary malignancy—an angiosarcoma of her chest wall—with the aim of controlling haemorrhage which is making her anaemic. Miss Mae speaks in an unusual pattern and you struggle at times to understand what she says. Your lack of comprehension appears to frustrate Miss Mae but she begins to speak more slowly, a consideration for which you thank her. Breast cancer, her primary malignancy diagnosed three decades prior, is metastatic to her lungs and her right humerus. Miss Mae, with significant haemorrhage at least twice each day and with fatigue from radiotherapy, says she feels terrible. 'I've nothing left. Nothing. But I'm not ready to die!' says Miss Mae when you meet her. Miss Louise sits behind her

[1] McCorkle's essays in *Cancer Nursing* are accessible at:
    https://journals.lww.com/cancernursingonline/pages/author.aspx?firstName=Ruth&lastNam e=McCorkle

sister, ramrod straight but with tears coursing silently down her face. You ask if Miss Mae is uncomfortable or in pain. She responds vigorously, saying 'No, the lovely doctors make sure I have not a moment in which I am uncomfortable. They don't know me, but they are on a first name basis with my pain!' Her sister shakes her head back and forth, implying some disagreement with what Miss Mae is expressing. 'No' says Miss Mae, 'I have nothing left in me. Death is coming but I don't have to welcome it'.

Your work to establish a therapeutic relationship with Miss Mae and her sister Miss Louise becomes paramount. Considering what Miss Mae told you without much prompting, you reflect to her that you would like to help understand what living until she dies means for her. Miss Mae speaks about her fears about being alone 'when it all ends', her love for her sister, and that she dislikes hospitals because she thinks she must be a good patient and 'not me, myself'. Miss Louise joins in now and the three of you talk, with some probing from you, about how Miss Mae lived her life, what she hopes for her death, and where she envisions staying at the end of her life. Miss Louise says, with Miss Mae nodding affirmatively, that her sister was 'special' growing up and did not learn easily in school. She left school early and took in work sewing. As she grew older, Miss Mae sometimes tried to work outside her home but never did so for long. She relied on what her siblings—all of whom except for Miss Louise are now dead—gave and eventually willed to her to 'make ends meet' as Miss Louise says.

Speaking together for over an hour, you identify that Miss Mac is strong minded and typically avoids any delay when she makes a decision. She prefers one to one interaction 'I'm not a social butterfly, like this girl here' Miss Mae says of herself and her sister. However, she speaks repeatedly about not wanting to be alone when 'the time comes', referring to her own death. You develop a plan with Miss Mae and Miss Louise where Miss Louise moves into the larger family with her sister so that Miss Mae receives home palliative care services along with support from her church's parish nursing team. Her home care includes nursing, physiotherapy, social work, volunteer caregiver support and personal care. Her sister and she are both older and live in constrained financial circumstances. You suggest connecting the social worker with the parish nurses to help locate resources for food and meal preparation. You arrange transport home for them as Miss Louise calls the chair of their parish nursing team. At the close of your meeting, you tell Miss Mae and Miss Louise you will call them in 2 days' time to ask how the plan is evolving and what further needs you might address. You also ask Miss Louise if she wishes to begin talking about the support she imagines she might want in her bereavement.

Reflective Exercises
- Begin examining your own attitudes toward ageing and unknowing ageism by taking the World Health Organization (WHO) Attitudes Toward Ageing Quiz (https://www.who.int/ageing/features/attitudes-quiz/en/) and then reflect on why you answered the questions in the way that you did. Then reread the practice example and reflect on how you think ageism may play out in similar situations for palliative and end of live care in your practice.
- Understandings of palliative and end of life care vary widely. Reflect on how you define these terms and why you do so. Consider how your practice site or agency uses these terms, if at all. Finally, reflect on how the definitions provided here support developing your practice.
- Try regular reflective writing or other reflective mechanism to contemplate your professional and personal experiences in palliative and end of life care. Use the key words and maxims highlighted in this chapter as signposts in your reflections.

Practical Tools
In addition to reflecting on maxims highlighted here, consider the following tools to support palliative and end of life care with older people

- When prognosis becomes a focus, consider the surprise question where a clinician asks themselves 'would I be surprised if this older person is no longer alive in 1- or 2-years' time?' is the most common trigger for referral for formal palliative care services. A 2-year time frame is often most used with older people who are multimorbid and living in their community [15].
- When considering home care, examine the Life Space Assessment. It is easily employed in practice as an assessment for home care needs and suggests dimensions of prognosis [16, 17].

10.4 Taking Your Studies Further

Several topics noted in this chapter offer possibilities to extend examination of palliative and end of life care in valuable directions. Ageism is pervasive in healthcare and worth studying in detail. Two current volumes address ageism quite comprehensively. They are Contemporary Perspectives on Ageism, edited by Ayalon and Tesch-Römer (open access and free to use at https://link.springer.com/book/10.1007%2F978-3-319-73820-8) and Ageism: Stereotyping and Prejudice against Older Persons 2nd edition, edited by Nelson (ISBN: 9780262533409).

Social death is an unfamiliar construct for many nurses and therapists. Borgstrom provides a lucid review of social death in a paper for *QJM: An International Journal of Medicine* (doi: https://doi.org/10.1093/qjmed/hcw183). Salutogenesis is often implicitly understood by nurses and therapists, making further study beneficial. The Handbook of Salutogenesis, edited by Mittelmark and colleagues, is a valuable resource (open access, available at https://link.springer.com/book/10.1007/978-3-319-04600-6).

Lastly, palliative rehabilitation is rising in prominence and offers possibilities to enhance palliative and end of life care. Among the resources available is a chapter entitled <u>*Rehabilitation in Palliative Care*</u> authored by Tiberini, Turner, and Talbot-Rice in the <u>Textbook of Palliative Care</u> (ISSN 3319317385).

10.5 Summary of Main Points

In this chapter, palliative and end of life care exist on a continuum where end of life care is palliative care near and at the time of death. End of life care may sometimes only be appreciated in hindsight, after death and during bereavement. Estimations of time to death are notoriously inaccurate and older people live with frequent multimorbidity and with proximate mortality. The imaginary of prognosis makes palliative care, defined without reference to prognosis or diagnosis, far more relevant to older people and our ageing world. Commonplace medicalisation of death risks limiting scope of and access to palliative and end of life care. Ageism threatens quality of all care including that which is palliative and provided at the end of life. Nurses and therapists hold paradigms that balance medicalisation and ensure palliative and end of life care are centred on the older person. Knowing the person and using maxims to guide palliative and end of life care ground that care in therapeutic relationships. Palliative rehabilitation offers utility in addressing hopes and fears with focus on function and comfort.

10.6 Suggested Reading and Resources

Center to Advance Palliative Care https://www.capc.org/

Lancaster University's International Observatory on End of Life Care https://www.lancaster.ac.uk/health-and-medicine/research/ioelc/

Palliative Care Australia's Resources Page https://palliativecare.org.au/resources

Royal College of Nursing End of Life Resources Page https://www.rcn.org.uk/clinical-topics/end-of-life-care/professional-resources

The Palliative Hub - Professional http://www.professionalpalliativehub.com/

World Health Organization's Palliative Care Page https://www.who.int/palliativecare/en/

World Health Organization's Global Atlas of Palliative Care at End of Life https://www.who.int/nmh/Global_Atlas_of_Palliative_Care.pdf

References

1. Hall LK (2017) Rehumanizing birth and death in America. Society 54(3):226–237
2. Pollock K (2015) Is home always the best and preferred place of death? BMJ 351:h4855
3. Walrath D, Lawlor B (2019) Dementia: towards a new republic of hope. Lancet 394(10203):1002–1003
4. Tiberini R, Turner K, Talbot-Rice H (2019) Rehabilitation in palliative care. In: MacLeod R, Van den Block L. (eds) Textbook of Palliative Care. Springer, Cham. https://doi-org.proxy.library.upenn.edu/10.1007/978-3-319-77740-5_34
5. Gullette MM (2018) When my mother wanted to die: the neglected issues of ageist undertreatment. Tikkun 33(3):6–9
6. Cary LA, Chasteen AL, Remedios J (2017) The ambivalent ageism scale: developing and validating a scale to measure benevolent and hostile ageism. The Gerontologist 57(2):e27–e36
7. Cottrell L, Duggleby W (2016) The "good death": an integrative literature review. Palliat Support Care 14(6):686–712
8. Öhlén J, Reimer-Kirkham S, Astle B, Håkanson C, Lee J, Eriksson M et al (2017) Person-centred care dialectics—inquired in the context of palliative care. Nurs Philos 18(4):e12177
9. Kagan SH (2017) Balancing the problem list with an advantage inventory. Geriatr Nurs 38(2):157–159
10. Sarton M (1989) After the stroke: a journal. WW Norton, New York
11. Win R (2019) The salt path. Penguin Random House, London
12. Benoliel JQ, McCorkle R (1978) A holistic approach to terminal illness. Cancer Nurs 1(2):143–150
13. McCorkle R (1981) A good death. Cancer Nurs 4(4):267
14. McCorkle R (In Press) Trusting the GPS: going home. Cancer Nurs
15. Lakin JR, Robinson MG, Obermeyer Z, Powers BW, Block SD, Cunningham R et al (2019) Prioritizing primary care patients for a communication intervention using the "surprise question": a prospective cohort study. J Gen Intern Med 34(8):1467–1474
16. Baker PS, Bodner EV, Allman RM (2003) Measuring life-space mobility in community-dwelling older adults. J Am Geriatr Soc 51(11):1610–1614
17. Kennedy RE, Sawyer P, Williams CP, Lo AX, Ritchie CS, Roth DL et al (2017) Life-space mobility change predicts 6-month mortality. J Am Geriatr Soc 65(4):833–838

Self-Neglect and Loneliness in Older Age

11

Lesley Hayes and Christine Cartwright

Contents

11.1   Learning Objectives

This chapter will provide you with the knowledge about how to:

- Understand key issues that can contribute to self-neglect and the effect it might have on a person's health and well-being.
- Understand key issues that can lead to loneliness and isolation and the effect it might have on a person's health and well-being.
- Develop awareness of how loneliness, social isolation or self-neglect can be assessed and addressed.

L. Hayes (✉) · C. Cartwright
School of Health and Social Care, Staffordshire University, Stafford, UK
e-mail: l.a.hayes@staffs.ac.uk; christine.cartwright@staffs.ac.uk

© Springer Nature Switzerland AG 2021
W. McSherry et al. (eds.), *Understanding Ageing for Nurses and Therapists*,
Perspectives in Nursing Management and Care for Older Adults,
https://doi.org/10.1007/978-3-030-40075-0_11

11.2   Introduction

This chapter explores the two distinct yet related concepts of self-neglect and loneliness/social isolation in the context of vulnerability. The section exploring self-neglect considers what self-neglect is, the range of contributing factors and its impact on health and well-being. Best practice when working with those considered to self-neglect is presented and the relationship with vulnerability and safeguarding is also explored. The section on loneliness explores the complex relationship between loneliness and isolation and begins to identify how it can be identified and addressed within a therapeutic relationship with clients. Tools for assessing loneliness are also considered.

11.3   Self-Neglect

11.3.1   Understanding Self-Neglect

Self-neglect is commonly considered to be both complex and challenging and the term itself can conjure up a wide range of emotions such as shame, embarrassment or disgust. However, the varied and sometimes subtle presentation means the characteristics of self-neglect are not necessarily easily recognisable or identified by practitioners [1] although it has been recognised for many years (e.g. [2]). Despite this, it has been comparatively under-researched, and although this means the characteristics and causes are not fully understood [1, 3] it has been found to be more commonly associated with older age [3, 4].

Although definitions of self-neglect vary, due in part to the individualised presentation, there are common elements that are associated with it. Braye et al. [5] for example note the lack of clear definition but identify three overlapping areas of self-neglect. These include a person's lack of self-care, neglect of their environment and refusal of services that would help address these. Consequently, self-neglect may include struggling with self-care through hindered capability or intention, and not providing oneself with sufficient or appropriate food, hydration, personal cleanliness, medication, clothing or a safe living environment [1, 3, 6]. The safety of the living environment may be compromised with elements of hoarding or squalor. There may also be disconnected essential services such as water or gas and property disrepair such as broken windows or leaking roofs. Self-assessment of need and acceptance of help from others may also be declined or accepted only intermittently [6]. Consequently, the emphasis currently is on deficit, what is missing, and the failure to provide self-care in these areas either due to inability or choice [1].

11.3.2   How Does Self-Neglect Affect the Individual?

Despite difficulties in defining self-neglect, authors have found strong evidence of it having a negative impact on the health and well-being of individuals, with studies consistently showing increased morbidity and mortality. Those who are identified as self-neglecting have been found to be more likely to have physical and mental health multi-morbidities such as diabetes, dementia, or depression and these may be untreated or inadequately treated [3]. Nutritional deficits which may be associated with poor nutritional intake have also been identified and may have further impact on the physical and mental health of the person [1, 3]. Likewise, dementia with its impairment of function, and depression have also been associated with self-neglect [1, 3]. An increased risk of death is also seen in those who are considered to self-neglect [1, 3]. Burnett et al. [3] report on studies that highlight this to be at least double compared to none self-neglecting adults.

Many of the elements associated with self-neglect such as hoarding or squalor cannot be readily seen in clinical areas [3]. Consequently, self-neglect may be more commonly identified within social settings, so emphasising the need for cohesive functioning of the wider multidisciplinary team (MDT) as the scenario below illustrates. Yet, as there are a wide range of factors and characteristics, it may be that self-neglect will never be definitively defined [1] and that individuals and teams will always develop their own intuitive sense of what constitutes self-neglect. Such tacit knowledge could potentially hinder communication with others within and across services and it is essential that this is addressed within teams. This could be achieved by ensuring more detailed assessments and MDT working.

Self-neglect because of its personal impact is associated with risk and concerns of harm. Yet, it can be challenging, as those who are identified as self-neglecting may also not engage with supportive services, or do so intermittently making a positive outcome difficult to achieve. Given self-neglect inherently has a negative impact on health and well-being, as identified above, it is also counter to positive ageing. It is essential therefore that practitioners are aware of the circumstances in which self-neglect may be evident and of the mechanisms by which they can address self-neglect in order to mitigate/ameliorate its impact.

> **Reflective Questions: Self-Neglect**
> Levi is 84 and lives independently. He finds it difficult walking and uses a wheelchair both inside and outside his home. He has difficulty looking after himself and doesn't want help from family or services. He rarely washes or changes his clothes and there is a large volume of rotting food in the kitchen and lounge. You are asked to visit Levi and to assess his needs. What concerns do you have about Levi and how do you feel about caring for him? How would you work with Levi to address these concerns?

One significant risk factor for self-neglect noted by Touza and Prado [6] is reduced social resources, including social engagement and informal social networks. Social isolation whereby people don't interact with others in the community has also been found to be associated with self-neglect [3]. Whether one largely causes the other isn't known. It is however likely that self-neglect leads to people disengaging socially from others. This means there may be a lack of support should it be needed, which could also lead to a decline in health and well-being, for example if health declines or people become less able with age-related changes. The lack of support networks may therefore result in people's health and well-being declining further.

This suggests that fostering and maintaining social connections may also help mitigate against self-neglect. If this is the case, the same approaches advocated to address loneliness and isolation could also prove beneficial when working with those considered to self-neglect, when considered as part of the wider support as discussed below.

11.3.3 Best Practice

It is essential to work across the multidisciplinary team (MDT) in order to successfully identify the relevant issues/concerns and to provide individualised and appropriate support for the person identified as self-neglecting [6]. Engagement however is difficult when the person does not want contact with services. This highlights the importance of a relational approach which helps develop trust and to create a relationship where positive contacts may become more likely. This requires ongoing regular contact and monitoring to establish a positive link.

The Social Care Institute for Excellence (SCIE) [7] however outline a wide range of barriers to good practice which extend beyond the persons' characteristics and their immediate needs. These include organisational aspects such as uncertainty around who takes responsibility for care delivery or service emphasis on shorter term provision due to funding constraints. These make relational based approaches and effective delivery of care more difficult and increase the risk of people 'falling through the net'. As a result, SCIE's good practice strategy aims to overcome these risks by recommending clear collaboration across agencies (multi-agency working) and developing agreed responses to self-neglect and pathways of care both within and across agencies. They also recommend a longer-term relationship-based approach to supporting the person concerned. On an individual level therefore, they indicate that individualised and collaborative support that aligns to the persons wishes, and which respects their perspective and goals is essential. The relationship is important as trust and ongoing connection can facilitate change, but people also need reassurance, patience and to have trust in the practitioner. The practitioner therefore needs to be empathetic and non-judgemental in order to ensure a positive relationship can begin to develop and where change may eventually be effected. This may require service providers to accept that change may be minimal or not occur, whilst simultaneously striving to find solutions and encouraging the person to identify potential alternatives to their current situation. So, given the risks associated with self-neglect, it is also important that there is ongoing risk assessment and risk management. Solid, effective and empathetic communication is therefore key. SCIE [8] usefully identify a number of practical actions encapsulating all these elements with the aims of reducing risk and of achieving a positive outcome. These include:

- Undertaking assessments of risk, mental health and capacity,
- Referral and signposting to other services such as occupational therapy, decluttering services or property maintenance services where appropriate,
- Potentially referring to counselling or therapy where other issues such as drug or alcohol dependency exist,
- Potentially talking to family or linking the person with others for peer support,
- Working with a wide range of organisations where appropriate such as environmental health, fire services or housing.

The overarching approach emphasises individualisation and is one that is values based and person centred. SCIE thus highlight the need to know the person and to understand what might be contributing to their self-neglect alongside providing respectful care that has characteristics such as being supportive, non-judgmental, empathetic, reassuring and encouraging change. This approach therefore leans towards an asset-based approach where autonomy is inherent, and interaction is positively framed in order to increase the likelihood of a positive outcome for the person. However, culturally sensitive strategies should be employed to ensure support meets the needs of the individual.

Although self-neglect doesn't automatically align with the idea of positive ageing, taking on some of the associated principles such as emphasising ongoing health and well-being could help guide the nature of and the way in which support is provided. One way of shifting to a more positive way of working with service users is to adopt a strengths-based approach as advocated by Britten and Whitby [9]. This includes recognition of individual strengths and those of their community such as friends and family. Assessment of risks, and strengths and their consideration in planning care will facilitate development of a person-centred approach and plan. The tools Britten and Whitby [9] provide encourage an holistic risk assessment including assessment of physical health, mental health and social well-being.

Practice Example: Self-Neglect

Rowena is an older woman who has lived in the local community for many years, she has a minimal pension and struggles with covering living costs. She shares her home with her cousin John but they tend to live separate lives. Rowena has fallen and John has raised the alarm with neighbours who immediately rang the paramedics/emergency services. On entering the house, the paramedics are concerned about the condition of the house and at how unkempt Rowena appears. They also realise during their physical assessment that there is no heating and the cooker isn't working. With consent Rowena is transferred to hospital as the assessment suggests Rowena may have broken her hip. Once Rowena is transferred to hospital the paramedic staff raise safeguarding concerns with regard to Rowena's home circumstances and her physical appearance. Once raised, an investigation is commenced. In the hospital setting an assessment is carried out including taking vital signs and a full physical assessment. Further investigations including an x-ray and bloods are ordered. Rowena was found not to have broken any bones and her bloods are not deranged. A comprehensive skin assessment leads to nurses identifying a pressure wound on her left buttock. This is assessed and an appropriate dressing applied to facilitate the creation of an effective wound healing environment. Planning for discharge includes discussion with Rowena about service support on returning home. She agrees to referrals to social services and community nurses in the short term. The community nurses lead on Rowena's support and care at home and work closely with other professionals and third sector organisations to support her. Once at home Rowena decided she didn't want support workers or social care staff to visit, but she did have a good relationship with one nurse, Sam, and would allow them to visit and to sometimes change her dressing. Over time, Sam became the key link for Rowena and through ongoing contact was able to develop Rowena's trust in her. Consequently, Rowena later agreed to Sam liaising with other services to get her heating repaired. Rowena didn't want any support for cleaning the house but was concerned about not being able to cook. When discussing this with Sam, Rowena said she had been finding it difficult to use the cooker but did like a good nutritious meal. Options were explored and Rowena felt that using a microwave and having pre-cooked, reheatable meals delivered would be a good option for her at the moment. Rowena agreed to Sam organising this on her behalf as she doesn't have a telephone.

This relationship-based approach to care meant Sam continued to visit Rowena and together they were able to review Rowena's circumstances on an ongoing basis. Through ongoing contact, Rowena began to see that she had strengths individually and in friends and family who supported her. She was slowly able to acknowledge these and to identify how she could make changes in her life by drawing on her strengths and support from others to help maintain and further develop her overall health and Well-being. Rowena's situation shows the importance of communication across teams and of a person-centred with the client.

11.3.4 The Relationship with Vulnerability

Pereira [10] considers vulnerability as applying to groups of the population who are at more risk of harm than the wider population. This does not however determine that all members of the group are vulnerable, and it is important to ensure that people are also seen as individuals [10], including when they are older adults who are considered to be self-neglecting.

The majority of research looking at self-neglect has taken place in America, where it is the largest form of elder abuse reported to Adult Protective Services [1]. More recently in England, due to rising concerns around its negative impact, self-neglect has also been formally recognised within the Care Act (2014) in relation to adults. Consequently, it is often strongly entwined with the concept of safeguarding (see [9]) thus formally linking self-neglect with the concept of vulnerability. There is therefore an emphasis on the risks, or of not having adequate safeguards when considering vulnerability in older adults [11]. Unfortunately, such emphasis can result in care and support that emphasises reduction of risk in order to safeguard the individual, and in doing so this can result in neglect of the right to autonomy [11]. The need to balance these, and to take managed risks is challenging and magnified in self-neglect where the outcome can be highly detrimental to the service user. Therefore, approaches which embed the principles outlined by SCIE [7] and Britten and Whitby [9] are essential.

11.4 Loneliness

When was the last time you felt lonely? What was the situation you found yourself in? Were there any presenting circumstances? What time of life was this? How did you feel? How long did this last for? These are questions that may encompass some of the issues around loneliness, it might be transient, occur at any stage of life, or be as a consequence of a life event, for example. Loneliness is being increasingly recognised as a concern for all ages, it can have health, social, and psychological implications. Here we are focusing on how loneliness can affect older people and their well-being.

Older people may become lonely in later life and this may be as a consequence of changes in life's course and events which have an effect on the person's ability to make, sustain and maintain valued friendships and relationships. Societally there may be the prevailing stereotypes of older people as a homogenous group naturally being lonely purely by virtue of their status [12] which could obscure the reality of the individuals' experience of loneliness.

Loneliness and isolation are themes commonly used interchangeably, seen to be an individual's emotional response to their own circumstances, creating concern and risk in both the mental and physical health of older people. These are now seen as two distinct and complex concepts. Defining these concepts can lead to debate and blurring of boundaries, however in simple terms both experience a lack or deficiency in their situation. Loneliness can be seen as an individual's negative emotional response to a perceived lack in the relationships they have or the relationships they would like, whereas isolation can be a physical reality of one's own remoteness in a community or lack of personal connections [13–15]. Individual factors such as age, gender, sexuality, ethnicity, and religious beliefs are not recognised as causes of loneliness. However, stigma, social issues, poor education, health issues, and poverty can all contribute to isolation.

11.4.1 International Perspectives

The World Health Organisation [16] acknowledged the importance and relevance of older people in society and their contribution to family life, the world of work and volunteering. The WHO, when looking at risk factors to mental well-being in older people, identified causal points such as physical health decline and frailty, but other challenges include a drop in socio-economic status, bereavement and difficulties such as isolation and loneliness.

Health and social care provision are focused on the needs of individuals, families and communities with specific health or social challenges. This can encompass holistic care approaches including the psychological, emotional, biological and social requirements of those groups. In Western societies, where capitalist political ideologies are a key feature, their populations are governed by life cycle activities including the statutory attendance of school for children, working in private or public sector industries for adults of working age and then an expectation to take retirement at recognised socio-economic age ranges. Increasingly, the themes of loneliness and isolation are becoming a significant concern from both a health and political perspective, especially in rich western countries.

In 2018, the Kaiser Family Foundation [17] carried out an international survey in loneliness and social isolation in the United States, the United Kingdom and Japan. The survey identified one in ten adults in Japan and over a fifth of adults in the United States and the United Kingdom felt they were often or always lonely. Factors arising from the survey documented the relationship between loneliness, and physical, mental and financial difficulties. Often those surveyed would report a negative event or change within the past 2 years contributing to their situation and there was debate around the influence technology has on loneliness and isolation. Bereavement rated the highest factor, then life changes including financial status, living situations, and health (severe and chronic long-term conditions).

In the United Kingdom, politicians have become increasingly concerned about the health impacts of loneliness; there has been a national campaign to raise awareness of loneliness such as the 'Campaign to End Loneliness' [18] and appointments at governmental level have created a minister for loneliness to oversee this issue. Investment has been made in two specific areas, namely healthy ageing programmes and to support those organisations who work to alleviate loneliness [19].

11.4.2 The Impact of Loneliness

According to Cacioppo and Patrick [20], there are serious health implications and impacts for those who identify as living with loneliness, which can include the chronic debilitating effects of stress on the immune system and cardiovascular system, as well as mental health issues including anxiety and depression. Ultimately there can be risks of suicide. Those living with dementia may find loneliness a factor in their illness, which can be twofold, with the deterioration of socialisation abilities as the illness progresses and the social withdrawal of others due to stigma or fear.

We are aware of the challenges of those who feel lonely and isolated, and the multi-faceted causes and contributing factors that affect them, so how do we recognise those clients, service users or patients who may experience these issues?

Reflective Questions
Spend a couple of minutes thinking about the people you have come into contact with and whether they appear lonely, do they have some of the indicators highlighted in this chapter? What is noticeable and what is said?

It is not always easy to identify those who are lonely by appearances, often it is by the self-report, the comments or behaviour of our clients. Identifying the person who is lonely is key, and there may be barriers to this, especially with older people, who may be from a culture of uncomplaining, being stoic and not comfortable disclosing personal issues. Society is built on ideas and values around relationships, cooperation, communities, belonging and acceptance, so it may be difficult to admit when a person feels lonely as they may perceive (incorrectly) it is because they are unworthy of friendship or companionship, or fear stigma [21]. To disclose feelings of loneliness can have significant self-concept issues, as we live in a society which celebrates autonomy, self-management and independence, and to fall short of one's own life expectations can create distress and disillusionment. Loneliness can also become a vicious circle, with the person who is chronically lonely losing their ability to become sociable and form the links and relationships they wish to develop [22].

11.4.3 Best Practice

The importance of developing a therapeutic relationship with clients cannot be underestimated, it can create trust, a sense of being understood, respect and wellbeing, this can assist you in establishing empathetic approaches to their care. This relationship can create the climate for discussion and space for disclosure. You may want to make gentle enquiry into the client's lived experience by asking some low-level questions such as:

- Have you ever felt lonely?
- When did you feel that way?
- How long did it last?
- What did you feel?
- What did you do about it?
- Do you feel that way now?

This may give the client permission to open up or consider these questions, as they may have not had an opportunity to express these experiences and feelings before. Having an opportunity to explore these issues and determine understanding of how this affects the person, it is important to establish a holistic assessment, taking into account their present life situation, health, mobility, home/living circumstances, finances for example. Ultimately, it is essential to be guided by the person and explore what would they consider helpful. Using tools such as the UCLA loneliness scale [23] may assist, informing a baseline of the situation as part of a holistic assessment and might clarify the client's experience however, it is the use of the information gathered from the overall assessment that will form person-tailored interventions.

Loneliness is not an illness, though lack of others in one's life may result in poor regulation of smoking and drinking habits, eating unhealthily for example, and much of its roots lie in the social aspects of a person's life [21, 24]. Working with people to overcome loneliness, interventions need to be considered in a sensitive and paced way. Admitting loneliness may create sadness and low self-esteem, so solutions may need to consider self-esteem and well-being factors. Working with clients to identify ways to reduce loneliness may be a progressive and staged intervention, where esteem and confidence building is an important first step, developing skills to manage stress and anxiety may be an area to explore, before looking at more direct social interactions. Encouraging clients to determine their own goals, discoveries of interests, former life roles and activities may be of benefit. Some local authorities and organisations have befriending schemes, volunteering activities, cross-generation activities promoting life skills to benefit other generations in the community, the use of digital and telecommunications, specialist focused activity groups such as Age UK's Men in Sheds scheme [13].

Reflective Questions
Loneliness
    Think about which groups of older people are affected by loneliness and how you might recognise loneliness within them.
    Following on from this, think about the obstacles that could prevent you from identifying loneliness in clients/patients/service users.
    Once loneliness has been identified it is important that this is addressed. What actions would you take to support a person identifying themselves as lonely.

11.5   Isolation

Isolation has been identified as physical remoteness and separation from others. This can cover all ages across the life span and cover a wide range of issues around social inequalities, access, poverty and health [21, 25]. Western industrialised societies appear to have increasing numbers of isolation, with a reduction in mixed generational families living together, higher rates of divorce and single occupancy homes, movement and migration for work, technological advancements reducing face to face contacts, as well as living longer with disease and illness [22]. Older people's risks of isolation are similar to other groups, including encountering mental and physical health problems, migrant populations, socio-economic factors and gender. Interestingly, according to a report by Public Health England and UCL Institute of Health Equity [25] older men experienced higher incidences of social isolation than women. This was attributable to males having less interactions on a regular basis with family members and friends. Poverty also had an influence on isolation, as affordability and access to transport, food, heating and social activities all were affected. Homes become a focal point for older people, where they have not only financial but emotional investment, memories and personal connections. There is a reluctance to leave homes, which hold such personal value and fears to avoid dependence and burden to others may be a feature. Frailty and lack of mobility will increase the risk of isolation. The solutions to these issues are complex, with a focus on societal changes in policy, community coherence and individualised support. All the factors to some extent will have an impact on the older persons' sense of isolation and in turn, loneliness.

Practice Example: Loneliness/Isolation

Stanley has moved into sheltered accommodation on a 3-month trial following the recent loss of his wife Sheila of 45 years. The accommodation is an independent-living flat on the first floor of a large complex (over 60 flats) on the outskirts of town, with 24-h assistive living. Both Stanley's children believe this is the best option for him, having a ready built community and will provide reassurance of 24-h help to keep him safe.

Stanley is an army veteran and when he retired from the armed forces he was reliant on Sheila for restoring his confidence and reintroducing him to civilian life. They were content with their home life, gardening and growing vegetables on an allotment together, being part of a small community with friends.

Stanley at 74 is fit except for some arthritis in his left knee, he is finding it hard to integrate into his new surroundings, find a routine and make new friends. Stanley's daughter, Sarah, is worried about him, as he had made numerous telephone calls during the night asking for help, he appears to have no motivation, taking no interest in things and complains of being bored, having no one to talk to. Sarah has contacted the medical Centre about her father's changes in behaviour and mood.

A holistic assessment would look at both Stanley's physical and mental health, ruling out any pathological causes. Stanley would benefit with a one-to-one discussion about what he sees as a cause of his distress. This would promote person-centred care values and an opportunity to hear without judgement, Stanley's point of view. Factors such as Stanley's bereavement, premature move from his home and memories of Sheila, eradication of his usual routines and activities, being part of an established social circle could be identified as factors contributing to his loneliness. Nolan et al.'s [26] relationship-centred care approach would assist the practitioner, Stanley and daughter to discuss issues, acknowledging their own perspectives, and to achieve positive outcomes to assist Stanley find solutions. Stanley disclosed he had agreed to the trial at the flat to reduce his children worrying about him being alone as he did not want to be a burden, but he was not happy and his grief was worsened by being away from the home and memories he had shared with Sheila. It was agreed for Stanley to return home and for a befriending agency to act as link to support him in the first instance, as he readjusts to home life.

As a health practitioner what factors do you feel have contributed to Stanley's situation?

Does moving to a new flat have any influence on Stanley's Well-being?

What strategies would you recommend assisting Stanley?

Would using relationship-centred care (Nolan et al.) be a useful approach?

11.6 Summary of Main Points

This chapter has explored self-neglect and loneliness, two key challenges in older age that are associated with vulnerability. Self-neglect and loneliness are complex and varied aspects, with a wide range of effects. Guidelines for best practice are broad ranging and require collaborative working. Such a multidisciplinary approach ensures that the wide-ranging needs are considered and that risk is subsequently minimised. It is clear that an individualised and relational approach is necessary when working with those who self-neglect and those who experience loneliness, taking on a strengths-based approach will facilitate positive ageing in this context.

11.7 Suggested Reading

Age UK works to address loneliness. Their web page on loneliness provides a range of demographics and numerous links to other relevant research and information: https://www.ageuk.org.uk/information-advice/health-wellbeing/loneliness/

Britten and Whitby (2018) have produced a book that focuses on assessment of those who self-neglect. They have produced an accessible account of assessment that balances the risks and strengths to create a person-centred approach to self-neglect: Britten, S and Whitby K. (2018) Self-neglect. A practical approach to risks and strengths assessment. Critical Publishing, St Albans.

Buka et al. (2016) explores a wide range of issues relating to vulnerability in older adults: Buka P, Davis M., Pereira M (Editors) Care of the Vulnerable Older People. London, Palgrave.

Braye (2018) has undertaken research into self-neglect alongside Michael Preston-Shoot. This link takes you to a presentation on working with people who self-neglect and includes a video that explores hoarding from the perspective of someone who hoards. http://www.hampshiresab.org.uk/wp-content/uploads/Suzy-Braye-Engaging-and-intervening-with-people-who-self-neglectand-what-works.pdf

Campaign to End Loneliness Connections in older age is a UK-based initiative. It provides ideas of actions that can be undertaken to reduce loneliness and offers a range of information sources and tools that can be used. https://www.campaigntoendloneliness.org/. The following source provides a range of information about loneliness: Campaign to End Loneliness (2016) The Facts on Loneliness https://www.campaigntoendloneliss.org/the-facts-on-loneliness/

Jo Cox Commission, (2017) Combatting Loneliness One Conversation at a Time: A Call to Action https://www.jocoxfoundation.org/. This explores loneliness in a UK context.

Nolan, M. R., Brown, J., Davies, S., Nolan, J. and Keady, J. (2006) The Senses Framework: Improving Care for Older People Through a Relationship-Centred Approach: Getting Research into Practice (GRiP) Report No 2. (available at) http://shura.shu.ac.uk/280/1/PDF_Senses_ (accessed by 3.9.10).

Positive ageing is a website that promotes approaches to ageing positively. They have identified a range of videos that explore different aspects of ageing: http://positiveageing.org.uk/videos/

Preston-Shoot (2018) has also worked with Suzy Braye. This link takes you to a presentation that explores self-neglect, including the need for the integration of relational approach: file:///C:/Users/lah3/Downloads/Michael_Preston_Shoot_Self_Nelgect%20(1).pdf.

Self-neglect.org is an American site which provides information and guidance for families and friends of people who self-neglect. It has a range of visual and interactive resources to facilitate understanding of self-neglect: https://selfneglect.org/

Skills for Care aim to develop a well-skilled adult social care workforce in England. It provides some resources relevant to self-neglect, which includes a useful workbook; it forms part of the care certificate and focuses on safeguarding. Home page https://www.skillsforcare.org.uk/Home.aspx; Safeguarding adults workbook https://www.skillsforcare.org.uk/Documents/Learning-and-development/Care-Certificate/Standard-10.pdf

Social Care Institute for Excellence (www.scie.org.uk). There are many useful social care related resources on this site. Social Care Institute for Excellence (SCIE) 2018) consolidates much of the current thinking relating to self-neglect and provides person-focused guidance around this. The site includes guidance around self-neglect and safeguarding. https://www.scie.org.uk/safeguarding/adults/practice/questions. Publications include the comprehensive document 'Self-neglect at a glance' (SCIE 2018) which includes an outline of best practice. SCIE also provide a range of related free online courses including: An introduction to the mental health of older people https://www.scie.org.uk/e-learning/mental-health-older-people; Challenges, dilemmas and positive approaches for working with older people in care homes https://www.scie.org.uk/e-learning/managing-risk-minimising-restraint; Interprofessional and inter-agency collaboration (IPIAC) e-learning course https://www.scie.org.uk/e--learning/ipiac.

Pioneer Network aims to foster positive ageing and to challenge outdated attitudes.https://www.pioneernetwork.net/old-age-appreciated-positive-aging-movement/. Their resources explore aspects such as ageism and culture: https://www.pioneernetwork.net/resource-library/

Washington State Department of Social and Health Services provides a brief overview of self-neglect and actions individuals can take to avoid it: https://www. dshs.wa.gov/altsa/home-and-community-services/self-neglect

References

1. Dong X (2017) Elder self-neglect: research and practice. Clin Interv Aging 12:949–954
2. Clark AN, Mankikar GD, Gray I (1975) Diogenes syndrome. A clinical study of gross neglect in old age. Lancet 305(7903):366–368
3. Burnett J, Achenbaum WA, Hayes L, Flores DV, Hochschild AE, Kao D, Halphen JM, Dyer CB (2012) Increasing surveillance and prevention efforts for self-neglect in clinical setting. Aging Health 8(6):647–655
4. Preston-Shoot, M (2019) Self-neglect and safeguarding adult reviews: towards a model of understanding facilitators and barriers to best practice. The Journal of Adult Protection 21(4):219–234. https://doi.org/10.1108/JAP-02-2019-0008
5. Braye S, Orr D, Preston-Shoot M (2013) A scoping study of workforce development for self-neglect work. Skills for Care, Leeds. Skillsforcare.org.uk
6. Touza C, Prado C (2019) Detecting self-neglect: a comparative study of indicators and risk factors in a Spanish population. Gerontol Geriatr Med. https://doi.org/10.1177/2333721418823605. Accessed 30 July 2019
7. Social Care Institute for Excellence (SCIE) (2018) Safeguarding adults in practice. Adult safeguarding practice questions. Published March 2015, Updated July 2018. https://www.scie.org.uk/safeguarding/adults/practice/questions. Accessed 30 July 2019
8. Social Care Institute for Excellence (SCIE) (2018) At a glance 71: self-neglect. https://www.scie.org.uk/self-neglect/at-a-glance. Accessed 24 July 2019
9. Britten S, Whitby K (2018) Self-neglect. A practical approach to risks and strengths assessment. Critical Publishing, St Albans
10. Pereira M (2016) Elder abuse and safeguarding vulnerable people. In: Buka P, Davis M, Pereira M (eds) Care of the vulnerable older people. Palgrave, London, pp 127–144
11. Davis M (2016) Theories of ageing and vulnerable older people. In: Buka P, Davis M, Pereira M (eds) Care of the vulnerable older people. Palgrave, London, pp 9–37
12. Pikhartova J, Bowling A, Victor C (2016) Is loneliness in later life a self-fulfilling prophecy? Aging Mental Health 20(5):543–549. https://doi.org/10.1080/13607863.2015.1023767. Accessed 14 Oct 2019
13. Age UK (2015) Evidence review: loneliness in later life. https://www.ageuk.org.uk/globalassets/age-uk/documents/reports-and-publications/reports-and-briefings/health%2D%2Dwellbeing/rb_june15_lonelines_in_later_life_evidence_review.pdf. Accessed 3 Nov 2019
14. Peplau LA, Perlman D (1982) Loneliness: a sourcebook of current theory, research and therapy. Wiley, New York. cited in Hughes ME, Waie LJ, Hawkley LC, Cacioppo JT (2004) A short scale for measuring loneliness in large surveys. Res Aging 26(6):655–672
15. Schirmer W, Michailakis D (2015) Loneliness among older people as a social problem: the perspectives of medicine, religion and economy, ageing and society. https://www.researchgate.net/publication/281675132_Loneliness_among_older_people_as_a_social_problem_the_perspectives_of_medicine_religion_and_economy. Accessed 14 Oct 2019
16. World Health Organisation (2017) Mental health of older adults. https://www.who.int/news-room/fact-sheets/detail/mental-health-of-older-adults. Accessed 13 Oct 2019
17. DiJulio B, Hamel L, Munana C, Brodie M (2018) Loneliness and social isolation in he United States, the United Kingdom, and Japan: an international survey. The Kaiser Family Foundation. http://files.kff.org/attachment/Report-Loneliness-and-Social-Isolation-in-the-United-States-the-United-Kingdom-and-Japan-An-International-Survey. Accessed 14 Oct 2019

18. Campaign to End Loneliness (2016) The facts on loneliness. https://www.campaigntoendlone-liess.org/the-facts-on-loneliness/. Accessed 3 Nov 2019
19. Bellis A (2019) Tackling loneliness. Great Britain, House of Commons Library. https://researchbriefings.parliament.uk/ResearchBriefing/Summary/CBP-8514#fullreport. Accessed 3 Nov 2019
20. Cacioppo JT, Patrick W (2008) Loneliness: Human nature and the need for social connection. W. W. Norton, New York. cited in Griffin J (2010) The Lonely Society Mental Health Foundation, 2010. https://www.mentalhealth.org.uk/publications/the-lonely-society. Accessed 15 Oct 2019
21. Griffin J (2010) The lonely society. Mental Health Foundation. https://www.mentalhealth.org.uk/publications/the-lonely-society. Accessed 15 Oct 19
22. Holt-Lunstad J, Smith TB, Bradley Layton J (2010) Social relationships and mortality risk: a meta-analytic review. PLoS Med 7(7):2–19
23. Hughes ME, Waite LJ, Hawkley LC, Cacioppo JT (2004) A short scale for measuring loneliness in large surveys: results from two population-based studies. Res Ageing 26(6):655–672
24. Victor C (2019) What works well for loneliness? British Society for Gerontology: ageing matters. https://ageingissues.wordpress.com/2019/09/10/what-works-well-for-loneliness/. Accessed 3 Nov 2019
25. Public Health England and UCL Institute of Health Equity (2015) Local action on health inequalities: reducing social isolation across the lifecourse. https://assets.publishing.service.gov.uk/government/uploads/system/uploads/attachment_data/file/461120/3a_Social_isolation-Full-revised.pdf. Accessed 10 Nov 2019
26 Nolan MR, Brown J, Davies S, Nolan J, Keady J. (2006) The Senses Framework: Improving Care for Older People Through a Relationship-Centred Approach: Getting Research into Practice (GRiP) Report No 2. http://shura.shu.ac.uk/280/1/PDF_Senses_. (Accessed by 3 Sep 2010)

Legal and Ethical Aspects: Elder Abuse and Safeguarding

12

Paul Buka and David Atkinson

Contents

12.1   Learning Objectives

The aims are to enable you to…

- Consider professional accountability and responsibilities of healthcare staff and others as well as the legal and ethical implications applicable.
- Define abuse in respect of *vulnerable* older people who may be at *risk.*
- Reflect on ethical implications and legal frameworks which support the healthcare and social environment and apply to them to practise through use of contemporary examples where safeguarding has not occurred.

P. Buka (✉) · D. Atkinson
School of Health and Social Care, University of Essex, Essex, UK
e-mail: pbuka@essex.ac.uk; datkinc@essex.ac.uk

© Springer Nature Switzerland AG 2021
W. McSherry et al. (eds.), *Understanding Ageing for Nurses and Therapists*,
Perspectives in Nursing Management and Care for Older Adults,
https://doi.org/10.1007/978-3-030-40075-0_12

12.2   Introduction

This chapter considers the definition of abuse and how to empower and support older people who are 'at risk' of abuse and current interventions for detecting and recognising and preventing elder abuse through safeguarding potential and actual victims. It establishes a link to key ethical principles and legal frameworks. The problem is complex and may be extensive. The primary focus point will be UK frameworks, and where this may be applicable to countries with comparable systems.

Readers are encouraged to engage in reflective activities, with application to practice. It is notable that a number of publications on Healthcare Law and ethics, medical ethics or similar titles have a limited reference to 'safeguarding'.

According to Maslow [1], safety is placed in the second tier in its hierarchy, indicating that after basic needs such as food and shelter, safety needs must be met if people are to progress to fulfil their potential. The hierarchy of needs may be disregarded or go unnoticed until it is too late, when caring for a vulnerable older person. Safety has long been paramount for different civilisations. Historically, it was clear that societies banded together for protection, while reinforcing this with the building of city walls and fortifications. In contemporary society however, there is every effort to ensure our own physical safety and security by having locks, bolts, CCTV and other personal safety measures to safeguard us and our property. Vulnerable older people are susceptible to domestic or institutional abuse and this may take other non-physical forms such as psychological and emotional aspects.

12.3   Ethical Issues

Several publications define the way we should act, both personally and professionally. This chapter applies the four Bioethical Principles of Autonomy, Beneficence, Non-maleficence and Justice [2], which are the bedrock of healthcare professional conduct. Autonomy is the *freedom to choose* a course of action, and the choices a person makes must always be rationalised when making decisions about their care, such as whether they have consented to treatment of any kind. Beneficence is about *doing good* which means – in all aspects of nursing and healthcare in the best interests of the person in their care, which includes following national and local policies on safeguarding. Non-maleficence is about avoiding or doing *no harm*—which on occasion may prove difficult to achieve as many treatments involve some degree of pain, e.g. an injection, however the harm should 'not be disproportionate to the benefits of treatment' (Buka in [3], p. 97) and justice is *being fair* which in a caring scenario means, avoiding favourable treatment for some, and a fair distribution of limited resources. This can also mean ethically and professionally, 'doing the right thing'. An example is the moral and professional obligation to tell the truth. This is the 'right thing to do' and if applied in all cases, this may be equated to 'being fair' [4].

12.4 Elder Abuse and Safeguarding People at Risk

The Care Act 2014 defines an adult at risk as, 'any person who is aged 18 years or over and at risk of abuse or neglect because of their needs for care and or support' [5].

Safeguarding in this area is central to care of older people at risk. The context may be in care homes, within hospitals as well as in the service user's own home. Vulnerability takes many forms, and can be classed as physical or psychological. With people living longer, a significant number of older people are likely to become more at risk due to the ageing process and hence may need safeguarding. 'Elder abuse' in respect of older people is common to vulnerable groups, and is defined as:

A single or repeated act or lack of appropriate action, occurring within any relationship where there is an expectation of trust, which causes harm or distress to an older person.
Action on Elder Abuse Bulletin (May–June 1995, issue no. 11), London, https://www. elderabuse.org.uk/aea-ni-what-is-elder-abuse

Several cases highlighting individual and institutional abuse related to the safety and well-being of vulnerable older people have come to light. An example was the Mid-Staffordshire debacle, resulting in the Francis Report [6]. This is explored briefly below.

Elder abuse may take many forms and the institutional contexts may be deep-rooted in the organisational culture and will require effective interventions in the form of safeguarding policies. It will be a challenge for staff, but the law protects whistle-blowers. It may be difficult to spot the signs of abuse. The data below shows that this is an international problem (Table 12.1). This was based on the best available evidence from 52 studies in 28 countries and this demonstrates the extent of elder abuse, WHO [7].

Table 12.1 Systemic reviews and meta-analyses

Type of abuse	Elder abuse incommunity settings (1)	Elder abuse in institutional settings (2)	
	Reported by older adults (%)	Reported by older adults and their proximities	Reported by staff
Overall prevalence	15.7	Not enough data	64.2% or 2 in 3 staff
Psychological abuse	11.6	33.4	32.5%
Physical abuse	2.6	14.1	9.3%
Financial abuse	6.8	13.8	Not enough data
Neglect	4.2	11.6	12.0%
Sexual abuse	0.9	1.9	0.7%

By kind permission of the WHO September 2019
WHO [7] https://www.who.int/news-room/fact-sheets/detail/elder-abuse

There are several versions of categorising which have been revised in order to meet modern needs and definitions of abuse. The World Health Organisation also outlines the following classification:

12.4.1 Classification of Abuse

- *Financial abuse*
  Includes having money or property stolen, being defrauded or 'scammed', being put under pressure in relation to money or other property or having money or other property misused.
- *Physical abuse*
  Includes assault, hitting, slapping, pushing, misuse of medication, restraint or the use of physical sanctions.
- *Psychological abuse*
  Includes emotional abuse, threats of harm or abandonment, deprivation of contact, humiliation, blaming, controlling, intimidation, coercion and harassment. Can also include verbal abuse, cyber bullying, isolation, unreasonable and unjustified withdrawal of services or supportive networks.
- *Sexual abuse*
  Includes rape, inappropriate touching, indecent exposure and sexual acts to which the adult has not consented or was pressured into consenting to.
- *Discriminatory abuse*
  Includes harassment, slurs or similar treatment because of race, gender and gender identity, age, disability, sexual orientation, religion. These are 'protected characteristics' under the Equality Act 2010.
- AGE UK, (2017) Factsheet 78 Safeguarding older people from abuse and neglect September 2017 https://www.ageuk.org.uk/globalassets/age-ni/documents/fact-sheets/fs78_safeguarding_older_people_from_abuse_fcs.pdf

Furthermore, a wider definition of abuse includes:

- *Organisational abuse*
  Includes neglect and poor care practice within an institution or specific care setting or in relation to care provided in a person's own home. This may range from one off incidents to ongoing ill treatment. It can be through neglect or poor professional practice as a result of the structure, policies, processes and practices within an organisation.
- *Neglect and acts of omission*
  Includes ignoring medical, emotional or physical care needs; failure to provide access to appropriate health or care and support; or the withholding of the necessities of life, such as medication, adequate nutrition and heating.
- *Domestic abuse*
  Includes violence, psychological, sexual, financial, emotional abuse and patterns of coercive and controlling behaviour during a relationship between

intimate partners, former partners who still live together, or family members, and honour-based violence.

- *Self-neglect*
  Most forms of neglect or abuse are perpetrated by another person and the law generally presumes there is a perpetrator as well as a victim.
- AGE UK, (2017) Factsheet 78 Safeguarding older people from abuse and neglect September 2017 https://www.ageuk.org.uk/globalassets/age-ni/documents/factsheets/fs78_safeguarding_older_people_from_abuse_fcs.pdf

Elder abuse may take place in institutions or on the home. Burstow [8] found that in 22 London homes, 24.5% of the residents were prescribed antipsychotics of which 82% were inappropriate.

12.5 Safeguarding People at Risk

The term safeguarding encompasses a range of considerations and measures that can be taken when caring for others—in this case, older adults. In the UK, 63% of adult safeguarding concerns are for people aged over 65, though only 3% of domestic abuse survivors are accessing Independent Domestic Violence Advisor Services (Age UK 2020).

The Universal Declaration of Human Rights 1945 emerged after the World War 2, with the aim to protect vulnerable people. These were adopted by what is now the European Union as the European Convention on Human Rights 1950 with the following key articles 2, 3 and 5, 8, 14. Elder abuse and the need therefore, for safeguarding has been recognised internationally as an issue:

> *Mistreatment of older people—referred to as 'elder abuse'—was first described in British scientific journals in 1975 under the term 'granny battering'*
>   UN, World Report on Violence and Health p135, 2002 https://www.who.int/violence_injury_prevention/violence/global_campaign/en/chap5.pdf

Subject to the Health and Social Care Act (2014), local authorities have a general duty to safeguard vulnerable adults who are at risk of abuse. Neglect arises when there is an omission or lack of care provision. As to the question why would the need for safeguarding vulnerable older population as compared to other vulnerable groups such as children (or victims of domestic violence, in general) be a priority? The facts speak for themselves as it is unfortunate that some institutional abuse of older people has been evidenced by several cases resulting in serious harm or death at the hands of healthcare professionals or family members who they trusted, who are supposed to protect them. This may have been perpetrated due to organisational cultural failures and/or inadequate safety measures. Examples are the Mid-Staffordshire Hospital [6], which highlights cases of poor care and neglect, and more recently the Gosport Memorial Hospital where more than 450 reportedly died due to unnecessary opioid use [9]. There have also been examples of a trusted GP carrying out abuse and carrying out euthanasia of vulnerable older people, *R v Shipman - [1999] All ER (D) 105.*

One key Recommendation of the Francis Report included, compassion as a way of combating abuse, and '… a shared positive safety culture requires: shared values in which the patient is the priority of everything done; zero tolerance of substandard care; empowering front-line staff with the responsibility and freedom to deliver safe care; recognising them for their contribution; and that professional responsibility is accepted and pursued' [6].

Furthermore, Section 81, Care Act 2014 creates a statutory duty of candour. Whilst there is no statutory definition of crimes against older people, nor legislation allowing for an increased sentence (such as in hate crimes), 20–25 of the Criminal Justice and Courts Act 2015, the Crown Prosecution Service makes it clear they are committed to prosecuting offences against older people [10]. A victim of abuse may litigate for damages in compensation for personal injury caused by such abuse. Additionally, prosecution by the Health and Safety Executive, under the Health and Safety at Work Act 1974 may also follow subject to Sections 2, which relates to the employer duty of care 'to ensure the safety of those affected in their premises' and 7'… the duty of the employee, for example if a member of staff had been employed when they knew they were under influence of drink and made a serious error of judgement impacting on the care of older people, and as a result they were neglected'. This places a duty of care on the employer and employees, respectively, to ensure that no person is harmed due to an unsafe environment or practices. This is applicable to care of all persons including risk of abuse of vulnerable older people.

In some countries, there is a statutory duty of care to protect those at risk through risk assessment and risk management for people with disabilities. It is even more important to safeguard and empower those who lack mental capacity (Mental Capacity Act 2005, Australian Law Reform Commission, Equality, Capacity and Disability in Commonwealth Laws, Report No 124 (2014).

The term 'safeguarding' includes a range of measures that should be undertaken within a caring environment when elder abuse is suspected or detected. The question arises as to who has the ultimate responsibility to safeguard vulnerable older people. The term 'at risk' is appropriate. It applies to needs/risk assessment and risk management and will be used more in the current context. It is everyone's duty to safeguard vulnerable older people and this duty ranges from family and friends, members of the public as well as healthcare professionals as required by legislation.

An employing organisation has a legal obligation to ensure that vulnerable people are not exposed to risk and is required by law to assess for risk. Since the Disclosure and Barring Service (DBS) was established under the Protection of Freedoms Act 2012, employers must ensure that their employees are cleared before they can take up employment.

The current checks required include a range of levels as follows:

- A basic check, which shows unspent convictions and conditional cautions
- A standard check, which shows spent and unspent convictions, cautions, reprimands and final warnings
- An enhanced check, which shows the same as a standard check plus any information held by local police that is considered relevant to the role
- An enhanced check of the barred lists (this shows individuals who may not work with vulnerable children and adults, and prevents individuals from employment in order to ensure safety of those at risk)
- GOV.UK https://www.gov.uk/government/collections/dbs-checking-service-guidance%2D%2D2

Individuals with a criminal record (for example, for sexual offences), in countries with similar systems, are placed on an offender's register; in the UK, those on the barred list are not allowed to work with vulnerable groups such as older people or children. There is a link between mental capacity and abuse, which is a key component, and goes to the heart of decision-making [11]. For vulnerable people with capacity, varying degrees of facilitation of decision-making will be required. If, however, a person lacks capacity, acting in that service user's best interests is the most appropriate option. This is not the case if there is pre-existing evidence of decision-making via a legal instrument such as a Power of Attorney which indicates a person's wishes whilst they had capacity.

The Mental Capacity Act 2005 provides for an assessment for mental capacity and empowers a patient in decision-making, (principles 1–3) and to act in the patient's best interests for those who lack capacity (principles 4and 5). The Mental Capacity Act (MCA) 2005 came into force fully on 1st October 2007 with a framework for the assessment, treatment and care of those who are deemed to have impaired capacity. The five key principles for supported decision-making are found in section 2.

Fundamental Human Rights may be breached under the Universal Declaration of Human Rights 1945. One such key area is article 5, Human Rights Act 1998. What happens when a service user lacks capacity? An Independent Mental Capacity Advocate may be appointed under the Mental Capacity Act 2005. They have a responsibility to support and represent a person who lacks capacity in making certain decisions. There is also a provision for an Independent Mental Health Advocate who has a similar role in supporting a person who is subject to the Mental Health Act 1983.

A criminal offence may result from ill-treating or wilfully neglecting anyone who has needs for care and support. An offence of wilful neglect and ill treatment is subject to the Criminal Justice and Courts Act 2015. (This update inserts new law as—s 44, Mental Capacity Act 2005).

Elder abuse involving physical, financial or sexual aspects may have criminal implications, for example, assault or sexual offences or theft are crimes and therefore reportable to the police. It may be more difficult to recognise, or for the victim to prove psychological abuse.

Reflective Exercise

Mrs. A is a frail, 80-year-old with dementia living in a nursing home where you work. You notice that when one nurse is on duty, Mrs. A is more agitated and distressed. This may be a coincidence but when as happens every time this nurse is on duty you suspect mistreatment of Mrs. A in some way. On one occasion you hear Mrs. A scream inside her room when this nurse is in her room, and you see the nurse shaking Mrs. A shouting, at her to be quiet. In view of what you have seen and the fact that Mrs. A is unable to protect herself, what would you do?

Are there any physical signs of harm to Mrs. A—Either from this incident or any other bruises or marks? What are the risks in not reporting this incident? How long has this been going on?

Mrs. A lacks capacity, with intermittently memory.

1. How do you manage and what are her human rights?
2. What is your role as a healthcare professional?
3. How would you ensure she is involved in any decisions regarding her care?
4. Are other residents at risk?
5. Are any protective measures in the nursing home working effectively, and if not, what should you do about it?
6. Identify the type of abuse.

This may amount to hate crime or ill treatment or wilful neglect by a care worker or care provider (sections 20–25 of the Criminal Justice and Courts Act 2015).

- Ill treatment or neglect of someone who lacks mental capacity
- Unlawful imprisonment
- Theft
- Fraud
- Domestic violence

(Age UK 2020 p. 16, adapted)

Reflective Exercise Tips

Is there anything else you need to consider?

If you are a professional in this situation, it is advisable to discuss the situation with your manager before deciding what to do, so the issue can be addressed as soon as possible. The statutory guidance states:

> No professional should assume that someone else will pass on information which they think may be critical to the safety and Well-being of the adult. If a professional has concerns about the adult's welfare and believes they are suffering or likely to suffer abuse or neglect, then they should share the information with the local authority and, or, the police if they believe or suspect that a crime has been committed. You should receive appropriate training based on agreed safeguarding procedures, so you know how to act in these types of situations. This is a requirement of service provider registration with the care quality commission.
>
> (Age UK 2020, p. 10)

Elder abuse may also mean breach of human rights. The legal framework for safeguarding older people is underpinned by the post-world war 2 Universal Declaration of Human Rights 1945. This was an international treaty in response to the human rights abuses during the Second World War. This resulted in the Nuremberg Trials and the Nuremberg Code (1947) was in response to this. The European Convention on Human Rights (ECHR) (1950) became the linchpin for human rights within the European Union. The UK, as a signatory, implemented this via Human Rights Act 1998. Human rights are fundamental to every citizen's welfare, requiring of every state and public organisation, a general duty, to ensure protection of individuals.

12.5.1 Key Articles of the (ECHR 1950) Human Rights Act 1998

- Article 3 of the Human Rights Act 1998
- *A* Prohibition of torture
- *No one shall be subjected to torture or to inhuman or degrading treatment or punishment.*

This means that victims of elder abuse may invoke their human rights in court against a healthcare provider. This does not exclude their right to litigate for compensation in cases of personal injury. The principle was applied in ***Sevtap Veznedarodlu v Turkey (App. 32357/97), Judgement of 11April 2000; (2001) 33EHRR 1412)*** where the court ruled that, the state has a responsibility to safeguard human rights was for all, including a victim of torture.

In a healthcare setting, this means that the clinician must not subject the service user to inhumane or degrading treatment. Under normal circumstances, it is a breach of this human right to override a patient's choice. There are however exceptions such as emergencies, those sectioned subject to the Mental Health Act 1983 as well as those who are subject to Article 5, European Convention on Human Rights

(ECHR) 1950 and under the Equality Act 2010, Deprivation of Liberties Safeguarding (DoLS)—the new Liberty Protection Safeguards (LPS) [12] (from 2018/2019).

- Article 8... respect for privacy and family life, which relates to patient or service user's choice if they have capacity. Clinicians are required to facilitate the autonomous decision making and empower the patient. This also applies for those with disabilities.
- Article 14, non-discriminatory treatment. The Equality Act 2010 applies. This applies to fair distribution of resources which may be scarce. It outlaws treating service users less favourably on one of the characteristics and this includes age, sexuality and discrimination.

In Common Law, the 'neighbour principle' or test came from Lord Atkins' judgement, 'You must take reasonable care to avoid acts or omissions which you can reasonably foresee would be likely to injure your neighbour. Who, then, in law, is my neighbour? The answer seems to be persons who are so closely and directly affected by my act that I ought to have them in [mind] when I am [considering these] acts or omissions', *Donoghue v Stevenson 1932, AC 562.* As applied, this means that a healthcare professional or carer owes a duty of care to ensure that vulnerable older people are not injured due to negligent actions or omission. In Tort Law they are entitled to litigate for damages. A criminal prosecution may also follow a criminal act, where physical harm is caused.

An older adult with mental capacity needs *may be at risk of abuse* or *neglect, and unable to protect themselves from either the risk or the experience of abuse or neglect,* and the Care Act 2014 has applied since April 2015. Section 1 of the Act requires a local authority to promote individual well-being in all it does, including 'protection from abuse and neglect'. Local authorities have a duty of care to establish adult safeguarding agencies and to lead adult safeguarding agencies. Such authorities should be the first point of contact for those who wish to raise concerns. Professional Codes of conduct, ethics and the law underpin a framework for decision-making.

Case: DL v A Local Authority [2012] EWCA Civ 253, [2012] MHLO 32, at p101
Elderly infirm parents living in own home subject to son's alleged threats and bullying—One parent lacking capacity under Mental Capacity Act 2005, the Court of Appeal, per Lord McFarlane '...the High Court can make orders to protect vulnerable adults with capacity under the MCA, if their ability to make decisions has been undermined through being under constraint, subject to coercion or undue influence, or otherwise prevented from making a free choice or giving real or genuine consent'

12.6   Taking It Further: Safeguarding and Patient-Centred Care

The Bioethical Principles [2], (above) which are endorsed by all healthcare professional Codes of Conduct establish an obligation for the healthcare professional to safeguard patient or service users who are at risk, focusing on the 'to do no harm' maxim. This should aim to promote safety for vulnerable older people in their care. The duty of care is not only in ethics but also in Tort law of negligence, there is a requirement for the professional to ensure that vulnerable older people in their care are not harmed by their negligent actions or omissions, ***Donoghue v Stevenson [1932] AC 562 House of Lords***.

Hate crimes and harassment, or public nuisances are committed against vulnerable older people, and police and public authorities may not always appreciate the impact on victims. This is a form of elder abuse. It is possible therefore that due to perceived inaction that victims may be reluctant to complaint as a result. The true extent of the problem therefore may never be known. One must ask the question: if current interventions are deemed effective, why do we continue to have cases of elder abuse, especially institutional ones, where healthcare staff are expected to follow policy? The Convention on the Rights of Persons with Disabilities (CRPD), (A/RES/61/106) was adopted on 13 December 2006 at the United Nations Headquarters in New York and *'aims to, all categories of rights apply to persons with disabilities and identifies areas where adaptations have to be made for persons with disabilities to effectively exercise their rights and areas where their rights have been violated, and where protection of rights must be reinforced'*

In the UK, the NHS Constitution (2015) applies to patient-centred care by which staff empowers and safeguards vulnerable older people. This would include empowering them to report any abuse. Unfortunately, in a few cases, vulnerable older people have been abused by healthcare staff in whom they placed their trust.

Practice Example 1
Mr. A, a 90-year-old man is admitted to an acute medical ward with a urinary tract infection. He is delirious, shouting and confused and aggressive and is demanding to discharge himself. A nursing staff member is allocated to him as he is at risk of 'escaping' and injuring himself. He is refusing treatment and frequently tries to leave the ward.
   Key issues

1. How to manage his ongoing and day to day treatment decisions
2. Does Mr. A have mental capacity to make decisions
3. What is the process for assessing mental capacity

Consider:

- Capacity, Autonomy & Informed Consent to treatment, Re C Judgement (below)—'Foolish' decision
- Art 5 Human Rights Act 1998 Deprivation of Liberties Safeguarding (changing to Liberties Protection Safeguards)
- What are the roles of the independent mental capacity advocate and independent mental health act advocate?
- How can advanced directives be used to protect vulnerable older people?

(Please see below)

Vulnerable older people who may not only have a physical condition but also lack capacity deserve to be afforded even more interventions and safeguarding through others advocating for them as they may also be subject to scams or embezzlement of financial or property interests.

Case: Re C (Adult, refusal of treatment) [1994] 1 All ER 819
Mental illness and a patient's capacity.

C diagnosed with paranoid schizophrenia and was detained in Broadmoor secure hospital. He developed gangrene in his leg but against medical advice, refused to consent to an amputation.

The Court upheld C's decision.

Legal principle: The fact that a person has a mental illness does not automatically mean they lack capacity to make an informed choice about medical treatment.

Patients who have capacity can make their own decisions to refuse treatment, even if those decisions appear irrational to the doctor or may place the patient's health or their life at risk.

http://www.gmc-uk.org/guidance/ethical_guidance/consent_guidance_common_law.asp

The roles of the Office of Public Guardian include safeguarding vulnerable people at risk by investigation of abuse by:

- Deputies appointed by the Court of Protection
- Attorneys appointed under a registered lasting power of attorney (LPA) https://www.gov.uk/government/publications/safeguarding-policy-protecting-vulnerable-adults

An Independent Mental Capacity Advocate (IMCA) may be appointed by a local authority for those who have no family members, next of kin or court-appointed representative. An Independent Health Advocate (IMHA) is an advocate who supports service users who come under the Mental Health Act 1983 framework, and who are under section.

Other ways of 'respecting the patient's wishes' are through the use of 'Living wills'. If properly drafted, they will have the legal effect of establishing this. With respect to advance statements, they can only inform and are expressions of a person's preferences such as where they would like to spend their last days. However, the second category advanced directives have more force in law as they categorically state their wishes such as 'do not attempt CPR'. They do not however have the legal authority to instruct or compel healthcare professionals to provide specific treatment courses.

Reflective Exercise 2

Mr. J is an 82-year-old, who is recently widowed who is a retired engineer with osteoarthritis. He has relatively modest means and been relatively healthy and self-caring after losing his wife. He is very much aware though since a recent hospital admission, he has become frail and more forgetful. He lives in a three bedroomed bungalow.

He has had carers in the past that he subsequently refused as they only came in for a chat and cup of tea and did not carry out his care properly. He appeared to have been neglected. Recently his 50-year-old alcoholic son has moved in (his wife died 3 years ago). The son is a divorcee who is now single and has a history of alcohol abuse. Neighbours, Jill and John have heard signs of arguments and cries for 'help' late at time night. When they asked Mr. J, if he was alright, he says he does not want to discuss anything and says it's a family issue.

The neighbours notice extensive bruising on his face and Mr. J tells neighbours he fell. He nevertheless admits that he has had altercations with the son. Mr. J has thrown the son out when this has happened before, but the son is always allowed to come back when he apologises.

What advice would you give the neighbours Jill and John?

If Mr. J refuses to cooperate what is the neighbours of duty of care in law and ethics?

Can the neighbours report this to the police?

All person who are healthcare professionals owe a duty of care to report this as safeguarding issue.

Neighbours owe a common law duty of care to also report this to safeguarding authorities or the police if they suspect that a crime has been committed.

Reflective Exercise 2 Tips

Consider your duty of care as defined in the Donoghue and Stevenson Case 1932 (above). If Mr. J refuses to cooperate, the neighbours still have a duty to raise concerns regarding vulnerable person.

1. If they suspect that a crime has been committed, Section 44 Mental Capacity Act 2005 (Ill treatment or Neglect of a Person Lacking Capacity)
2. Sections 20 and 21 of the Criminal Justice and Courts Act 2015 (Ill treatment or Wilful Neglect by Care Workers or Care Providers) apply

The problem of elder abuse appears to be clearly worsening with, 'around 10% of the population aged 65+ in the UK reportedly experiencing some form of abuse. That is around 1 million people'. HMICFRS [13] www.justiceinspectorates.gov.uk/hmicfrs.

12.7 Summary of Main Points for Learning

This chapter presents an opportunity for the reader to enhance their working knowledge of the legal and ethical aspects of elder abuse and safeguarding. It contains a number of examples and cases in order to provide a framework which a healthcare professional may use to support their accountability and responsibilities when dealing with or caring for an elderly client or patient. The chapter includes ethical and legal discussion from a UK and an international perspective, where appropriate, in order to illustrate the complexities and difficulties of these issues. We find that most of the issues are transferable to other Western countries with similar laws and societal challenges. This chapter may offer some guidance in the decision-making and reporting process when faced with actual or suspected cases of elder abuse or safeguarding issues.

Information and guidance are unfortunately still necessary even in the twenty-first century as the statistics, cases, and laws contained in the chapter clearly demonstrate. Whilst we may consider our society to be 'civilised' and that we are far removed from the harshness and brutality of the past, it is abundantly clear that wherever there are people, there will always be those individuals who will take advantage of vulnerable people, and sometimes abuse older people who are at risk. It is this very fact that the need for this chapter is evident, and it has been written in the hope that the information and guidance it contains will at the very least, mitigate the risk or consequences of elder abuse, by enabling healthcare professionals to recognise those at risk of, or have been abused and take appropriate action.

References

1. Maslow A (1954) Motivation and personality. Harper, New York
2. Beauchamp T, Childress J (2013) Principles of biomedical ethics. Oxford University Press, Oxford
3. Buka P, Davis M, Pereira M (2016) Care of vulnerable people. Palgrave, London
4. Ellis P (2017) Understanding ethics for nursing students (Transforming nursing practice series), 2nd edn. Sage, London
5. NHS England (2017) Safeguarding adults. https://www.england.nhs.uk/wp-content/uploads/2017/02/adult-pocket-guide.pdf. Accessed 1 Oct 2019
6. Francis Report p 1357, 2013. Report of the Mid Staffordshire NHS Foundation Trust Public Inquiry vol 3: Present and future Annexes, HC 898-III London: The Stationery Office
7. WHO (2017) Abuse of the elderly, Chapter 5. https://www.who.int/violence_injury_prevention/violence/global_campaign/en/chap5.pdf. Accessed 12 Aug 2019
8. Burstow P, Keep Taking the Medicine 2, p 4 (based on Oborne, C. Alice et al) (2002) An indicator of appropriate neuroleptic prescribing in nursing homes. Age Ageing 31:435–439; Q 12
9. Gosport Independent Panel (2018) https://www.gosportpanel.independent.gov.uk/media/documents/070618_CCS207_CCS03183220761_Gosport_Inquiry_Whole_Document.pdf. Accessed 22 Sept 2019
10. Crown Prosecution Service (2019) Hate crime. http://cps.gov.uk/publication/policy-guidance-prosecution-crimes-against-older-people. Accessed 10 Sept 2019
11. Cooper C, Selwood A, Livingston G (2008) The prevalence of elder abuse and neglect: a systematic review. Age Ageing 37:151–160
12. Liberty Protection Safeguards (LPS) (2019) https://www.qcs.co.uk/overview-of-the-liberty-protection-safeguards-frequently-asked-questions/. Accessed 10 Oct 2019
13. HMICFRS (2019) The poor relation the police and CPS response to crimes against older people. www.justiceinspectorates.gov.uk/hmicfrs. Accessed 30 Aug 2019

Cases

14. DL v A Local Authority (2012) EWCA Civ 253, [2012] MHLO 32, at p101
15. Donoghue v Stevenson (1932) AC 562 House of Lords
16. Re C (Adult, refusal of treatment) (1994) 1 All ER 819
17. R v Shipman (1999) All ER (D) 105
18. Sevtap Veznedarodlu v Turkey (App. 32357/97), Judgement of 11 April 2000; (2001) 33EHRR 1412

Statutes (UK)

19. Care Act 2014, Section 1
20. Criminal Justice and Courts Act 2015, Sections 20 and 21
21. Equality Act 2010
22. European Convention on Human Rights (ECHR) (1950)
23. Health Safety at Work Act 1974, Sections 3 and 7
24. Human Rights Act 1998, Art 3, Art 5, Art 8, Art 14
25. Mental Capacity Act 2005
26. Mental Health Act 1983
27. Protection of Freedoms Act 2012
28. Universal Declaration of Human Rights 1945

Recommended Reading

Mandelstom M (2019) Safeguarding adults and the law. In: An A-Z of law and practice, 3rd edn. Jessica Kingston Publishers, London

Barnett D (2019) The straightforward guide to safeguarding adults: from getting the basics right to applying the care act and criminal investigations. Jessica Kingston Publishers, London

MK Shankardass (2019) International handbook of elder abuse and mistreatment hardcover, Delhi. Springer, Jessica Kingston Publishers, London

Applying Critical Concepts: Clinical Governance, Quality, and Review to the Older Persons Context

13

Robert McSherry and Patrick Pearce

Contents

13.1   Learning Objectives

This chapter will provide you with the knowledge about:

- Why is clinical governance important when caring for older people in health and care settings.

R. McSherry (✉)
Department of Nursing, School of Health and Social Care, Staffordshire University, Stoke-On-Trent, UK

University Hospitals of North Midlands NHS Trust, Stoke-on-Trent/Stafford, England, UK

Professor VID Specialized University College Bergen/Oslo, Oslo, Norway
e-mail: w.mcsherry@staffs.ac.uk

P. Pearce
Independent Healthcare Governance Consultant, Yarm, Stockton on Tees, England

© Springer Nature Switzerland AG 2021
W. McSherry et al. (eds.), *Understanding Ageing for Nurses and Therapists*,
Perspectives in Nursing Management and Care for Older Adults,
https://doi.org/10.1007/978-3-030-40075-0_13

- Raising your awareness of sound governance principles and practices and how these should be applied, adhered to, and evaluated when caring for older people.
- Recognising, responding, and knowing how to escalate care concerns for both patients and staff.

13.2   Introduction

In this chapter, we focus on dispelling and disentangling some of the myths displayed by health and care workers surrounding the *'critical concepts: clinical governance, quality, and review'*. We refer to these as critical concepts because of the following reasons. They are associated with how individuals, teams, and organisations explore, apply, review, safety, governance, and quality principles in practice. Careful analyses of their effect on people, systems, processes, and the workplace culture and environment are paramount in ensuring quality improvement and change. They are the bedrock or foundations to all matters related to safety and quality in health and care. Finally, they are often described by some health and care workers as jargonised, dry, not relevant to me, divorced and/or detached from the real world of health and care. They are for managers, not frontline workers. We believe these myths exist because they are often inextricably linked to an individual's level of insight and awareness of these critical concepts:

- This subsequently impacts on their level of engagement and application of the critical concepts to improve and change practice.
- This is often inherently akin to one's attitude, belief, and values held surrounding the terms.
- This influences their behaviour and approach to how they engage or not in applying the principles they bestow in facilitating safe, quality, care, and services.

The chapter aims to demystify the rhetoric surrounding these critical concepts by unravelling the terms using examples from health and care practice and in identifying their relevance to the delivery of safe, compassionate, dignified, and respectful care for older people. We will also look at the importance of these in relation to health and care organisational structures, systems and processes, regulation, policy and guidance and leadership and management. Finally, throughout the chapter we focus on identifying your individual role and responsibility when caring for older people. This is imperative in ensuring the principles are understood and applied to facilitate safe, quality care in your health and care setting.

13.3   Why Is Clinical Governance Important When Caring for Older People in Health and Care Settings

It is crucial to acknowledge and celebrate the fact that worldwide people are living longer. For some older people these are happy and healthy periods and experiences of their life. Quality of life and experiences include living comfortably and feeling safe, having a secure home and place of residence, a safe community and circle of friends and family. It is associated with staying active and healthy along with having the physical and mental abilities to get out and about, an acceptable income, and access to leisure and local amenities for ongoing learning and sources of sound information.

However, longer lifespan does not always necessarily equate to a happier, healthier, and fulfilled period in one's life for all older people. Sadly, with age for some older people comes physical decline; having multiple-co-morbidities and long-term conditions, psychosocial issues; social isolation, loneliness, anxiety, and depression. Regrettably, despite the safeguarding controls and measures put in place to protect and keep safe some of our most vulnerable individuals in society, in the extreme of situations for some, there is the abhorrent experience of abuse: financial, psychological, social, and physical.

Alongside the above factors is the notice by the World Health Organisation (WHO) that 'by 2020, the number of people aged 60 years and older will outnumber children younger than 5 years' [1]. This significant demographic trend requires the world's health and care systems to respond too and prepare for, for several reasons.

Older people should be supported to retain a high level of independence and quality of life, and where possible, this should occur within their chosen place of residence. To avoid upset and any confusion in later life, older people [indeed all people] should be encouraged to talk about, and document their preferences in advancement of old age, and where they would like things to happen. It is about ensuring that appropriate health, care, and social systems and processes are in place to ensure that older people, those with and/or without the capacity and capability to make decisions about their life and preferences are supported to do so. Where this is not possible, this should be done in conjunction and discussion with their legal next of kin, guardian(s) and/or enduring power of attorney(s). Similarly, it is about engaging with older people and their families to co-design, co-produce, and co-deliver the building of new innovative facilities, premises, services and/or provisions that recognise and respond to the priorities of older people. It is no longer acceptable for health and care providers to presume what older people require. Health and care services should not marginalise or discriminate older people but firmly place them at the heart of any system and process design, delivery, and evaluation. It is about: celebrating age and ageing; safeguarding and protecting the special characteristics that accompany an older person; providing safe, compassionate, person-centred care and environments; recognising the rich tapestry of the individual and their life journey; and affording them peace, choice, dignity, privacy, respect, and a peaceful death.

Reflective Exercise 13.1
Before proceeding further, we would like you to think about what factors may affect you in providing safe, quality and compassionate care for older people. We would like you to particpate in the following exercice by refecting upon how this may impact on the care of older people. Please follow the steps below:

- Step 1: Fold an A4 piece of paper into four sections as detailed below:

- Step 2: Place the following labels and/or categories: Professional, Political, Societal and Economical, like the example shown below.

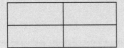

| Professional | Political |
| Societal | Economical |

- Step 3: Write down any thoughts and ideas that come to mind within the sections.

Do not overthink, note down what springs to mind and write your thoughts under the respective categories.

With regard to the Reflective Exercise 13.1 do not worry if your points are not similar and/or identical to ours detailed. This is because we all see the world and its challenges from different perspectives and points of view. Similarly, this may be the same within our own health and care organisation, and the workplace and environment in which we work. The important message to take away from the activity is to recognise and value the fact that we are all different but have a common goal and purpose in what we do. **That is, to provide the best possible care to our patients/ carers/work colleagues, and in creating the best possible workplace culture and environment for that to take place.**

In our opinion the drivers for safe, quality, person-centred health and care services can be distilled into four categories: **political, professional, societal, and economical** outlined in Fig. 13.1 below.

According to Fig. 13.1 **each category contains a multitude of complex and inter-related factors that may influence the delivery of health and care services for older people in either a positive and/or negative way.** In brief:

Political—drivers in our opinion appear to fall into two broad categories: **'changes in health and care policy' and 'care delivery systems'.**

Changes in health and care policy highlights the need for professional, organisational, and public accountability. This is realised by ensuring that health and care workers are made aware and informed of new and/or changes in any national, regional and workplace policies, guidelines, directives, and procedures, that they are implemented and adhered too. These may originate from professional bodies like the United Kingdom (UK) Nursing and Midwifery Council, General Medical Council, and Health Care Professionals Council. Regulators of care and services such as the, Care Quality Commission and Government Departments like, The National Health Service.

In addition, it is imperative for health and care workers to support their decision-making and actions with the most reliable sources of evidence. To achieve this, you *must* keep abreast of new and outdated legislation/policy/

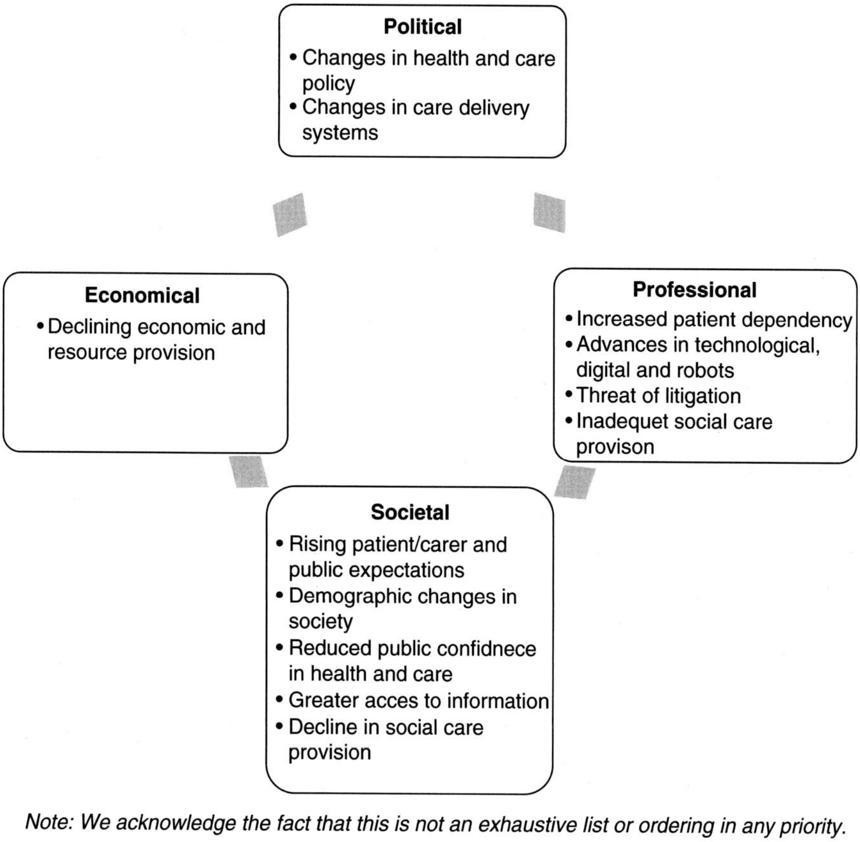

Note: We acknowledge the fact that this is not an exhaustive list or ordering in any priority.

Fig. 13.1 Drivers for safe, quality, person-centred health and care services. *Note: We acknowledge the fact that this is not an exhaustive list or ordering in any priority*

guideline, standards, and evidence. You *must* adhere to your codes and standards of professional practice, work within the scope, and remit of your professional and workplace contract of employment and job specifications. You *must* also have the necessary knowledge skills, competence, and confidence, to transfer policy, guidance, and evidence into your practice. To realise the later you must have access to the evidence-base for example, computers, databases and other technology and digital related materials and resources within the workplace.

Care delivery systems reaffirm the need for health and social care policy and decision-makers along with health and care workers, major stakeholders, patients, and the public to introduce systems and processes that meet the needs of the population. Care delivery systems should be designed to safeguard and protect those coming into contact with the services. They should also facilitate a workplace culture that empowers health and care workers to provide safe, quality care and service for older people.

Professional—primarily centres on health and care workers adhering to professional standards, regulations, policies, procedures, guidance, and laws. It is about ensuring decisions and actions are underpinned with evidence. *Evidence-based practice* in this context is:

> *an approach to decision making in which the clinician uses the best evidence available, in consultation with the patients, to decide upon the option which suits that patient best* [2].

Viewed in this way it is easy to see why evidence-based practice is inter-linked to '*accountability*'. In brief accountability (this is explored in more detail further in the chapter) is founded on the principals that we are all responsible for the decisions we make, the actions we take, as well as the consequences this may have on oneself and others.

Acknowledging the fact that older people have a complex diverse set of needs, requiring a set of diverse expertise. This is because health and care occur in a diverse range of settings and surroundings each having their own unique safety challenges. For example, caring for someone at home presents a set of challenges different to those when caring for an older person in hospital and/or residential/ nursing/care setting. Similarly, caring for an older person with dementia in any of these settings poses a different and diverse set of health and care challenges akin to safety for the individual and health and care workers.

Increased patient dependency and care left undone in both the health and care settings reinforces the need for health and care workers to have the necessary knowledge, skills, and competence to provide safe compassionate quality care. It is about recognising, valuing, respecting, and responding to the needs of the older person. An increasing patient dependency and staff shortages are resulting in skill-mix and workload issues where some health and care workers are providing suboptimal care and, in some instances, missing vital care procedures. These include for example, not responding to the deteriorating patient vital signs and not escalating accordingly and a failure to provide quality care and services. Having insufficient staff on duty can significantly compromise the delivery of safe, quality care and can affect the outcomes of care, i.e. safety, length of stay, mortality, patient/carer experience, effectiveness, and timeliness of care. Unfortunately, this has culminated with the term '*care left undone*', becoming more prominent across the globe [3].

The notion of care left undone is a real threat to health and care services for older people. This is because any reduction in younger adults to care for older people alongside a rising number of older people requiring care poses a real threat to workload, skill-mix and may compromise overall patient safety, quality, standards, and care. The authors feel that a health and care '*generational time bomb*' is just around the corner and requires immediate action by governments and health and care providers to overt a large-scale catastrophe. Any reduction in the availability of the health and care workforce and skill-mix could lead to a parallel reduction in the availability of expert services, facilities, and resources in the community, acute, social, and local authorities.

Internationally, inquiries, events, investigations highlighting failures in health and care for older people are occurring. Failures of both systems and people repeatedly happened where unnecessary and avoidable harm (never events), serious harm, and death occurred and is reported in the press and media. Recently in the United Kingdom, The Whorlton Hall Scandal of 2019. A privately run 17 bedded hospital providing care to vulnerable adults was investigated by the UK care regulator of reported 'abused'. The hospital was closed, and patients were transferred to other care sector services for their safety. Police investigations where potential criminal processions are could be made as still ongoing [4].

The Mid Staffordshire National Health Service (NHS) Foundation Trust scandal 2016. This major scandal between 2005 and 2008 was reported many times in the media and press, where it was estimated that due to the neglectful, harmful, and substandard care, between 400 and 1200 patients (many older patients) than would be expected for this type of hospital [5].

The South African scandal of 2017 was investigated where it was reported that nearly 100 mental health patients died due to neglect and maltreatment [6].

Threat of litigation. Regrettably, over the past two decades, we have witnessed a huge rise in the numbers of formal complaints, proceeding to litigation, made by patients and carers about hospital and community services. The cost to the National Health and Care Services of clinical negligence claims was £1.6 billion in 2016–2017. This is quadruple on the numbers for 2006–2007, according to figures from the National Audit Office. In the same time frame, legal costs for these claims have risen from £77million to £487million [7]. These rising costs, associated with litigation, are attributed to increased activity levels within health and care and the propensity to pursue a complaint to litigation because of the inflated compensations for negligence claims, if outcome can result in monetary gain. Complaints can be reduced, by ensuring that the care given to patients/carers is relevant to them and based upon the best available evidence.

Societal—factors have and will continue to play an enormous part in influencing the safety, quality, and standards in health and care. *These factors can be traced back to societal changes associated with rising public expectations and their lack of confidence in health and care services.* This is primarily due to a perceived decline in the provision of quality services and standards of health and care and the slow uptake of technologies, such as digital, computer, informatics, and data protection systems and processes. The public and health and care professionals themselves could be seen to have exacerbated these rising concerns, by involving the media, in reporting major clinical incidents and declines in the standards of services within the health and care services in which they are employed.

Globally, the public's growing lack of confidence in the health and care services could be attributed to the following: lack of financial investment, poor leadership, and management, or even, unsuccessful reform through government policy. We would argue that recent clinical disasters identified above have only served to shock the public into thinking that these are common occurrences, and that the overall standards and quality of service are poor throughout world. *In recent years, the advances in technologies and the easy access to information on the World Wide Web have resulted in the public becoming better informed, educated, and more interested in health, care, and policy-related issues.* This is evident by the upsurge in social movement activities, including media campaigns, people marches designed to influence policy and strategy through indirect actions and consequences. Examples include, save our hospitals campaigns, and patient and public involvement marches associated with care and neglect of services.

Health and care workers and the public themselves are now able to access information, research, evidence via the internet, regarding 'best treatment', interventions, policy guidance. As consumers of health and care, they are able to access the same information as any health and care professional. This empowers the public to seek specific information relating to their and/or family members' condition. This ability to access information (research, evidence), which was perhaps difficult to obtain previously, is fuelling the public's demands and expectations for safe, quality care as well as improvements in health and care systems and technology. *As a result and identified previously the public are not prepared to accept suboptimal standards of practice, resulting in a higher number of individuals and/or groups in seeking satisfactory outcomes through the courts.*

Economical—*'Our health and care needs are changing: our lifestyles are increasing our risk of preventable disease and are affecting our wellbeing, we are living longer with more multiple long-term conditions like asthma, diabetes and heart disease and the health inequality gap is increasing'* [8].

Considering the above it is not surprising that the burden of disease and impact on the quality of life, health and wellbeing of individuals continues to rise annually. Increasing life expectancy in parallel with rising *'multi-complexities'* (i.e. requiring care from more than one service at the same time such as medical, nursing, and social care). The latter coupled with *'multimorbidity'* (having several medical conditions some of which may also be a long-term condition, i.e. respiratory, cardiac, ophthalmological, etc.) of patients is growing exponentially. *The cumulative effect of these factors alone (not including the societal, professional, and political factors identified previously) has resulted in rising costs to accommodate these health and care trends and demands.* To keep pace with these rising demands and costs requires greater funding and/or redesigning of service provision. In some instances, the need for rationing, as well as the privatisation of a number of publicly funded health and care services.

The growth in health and care need and complexity, together with the expansion of care provision and services, have witnessed significant shifts in the leadership and management styles of health and care senior executives, managers, leaders, commissioners, and providers of care to address these rising demands and costs.

New terms like population health management (PHM)

is helping us understand our current [situation], and predict our future, health and care needs so we can take action in tailoring better care and support with individuals, design more joined up and sustainable health and care services and make better use of public resources [8].

The importance of having integrated joined up health and care services is imperative in order to address local population health trends and need. This type of integrated service leadership and management enables teams to focus on specific resources to accommodate and mitigate current and future needs. A strategic approach is required to specially focus on the increase in the rising population of older people and subsequent demands. These increased demands result in higher numbers of older patients being admitted with multiple needs. *This significantly impacts on the health and care workforce providers, who have had to change their patterns of health and care delivery, to accommodate this growing trend.* Some excellent examples include:

- Seven-day working, out-of-hour care services.
- Urgent and emergency care services.
- Continuing care services.
- Fragility services for older people.
- Video-conferencing and telephoning General Practitioner (GP) consultation.
- The establishment of acute medical, or surgical assessment units.

We have also witnessed the development of hospital recovery plans designed to maximise the use of acute and community beds and encourage integrated collaborative working between primary and secondary care. *These rising patient numbers and complex needs are increasing service demands, resulting in the urgent development of new ways of providing care* [9]. Some emerging initiatives include hospital and/or care at-home schemes designed to maintain patients in their own homes; Public and private sector partnerships (where acute illness is managed in hospitaland rehabilitation is continued in private nursing homes, until the patient is ready for discharge home).

We would argue that the cynics may suggest that these driving force behind such innovations above could be attributed to having reduced junior doctors' hours together with the possible consequences of the '*European Working Time Directives*' [10], and 'Brexit' (The United Kingdom leaving the European Union).

Health and care workers are rising to meet the challenges posed by the increasing numbers of patients with higher dependency needs, by developing new, creative ways of working. These include, for example, the introduction of emergency care, nurse practitioners, surgical care practitioners, and nurse consultants into busy and demanding clinical areas, like acute medical admissions and accident and emergency departments, in a drive towards improving the quality of health and care services.

13.4 Raising Your Awareness of Sound Governance Principles and Practices and How These Should Be Applied, Adhered to, and Evaluated in Your Practice

The evolution of **'clinical governance'** in England's National Health Service (NHS) can be traced to the white paper 'The New NHS Modern, Dependable' [11]. Originally coined by Sir Liam Donaldson it was defined as:

a framework through which NHS organizations are accountable for continuously improving the quality of their services and safeguarding high standards of care by creating an environment in which excellence in clinical care will flourish [12].

Following the UK government's initial definition of clinical governance, the term has become internationally recognised as a framework or **panacea for improvement and change** of the health and care systems and services. This is because it pulls together a whole range of organisational structures and departments by focusing on **the systems and processes with a strong emphasis placed on accountability associated with the maintenance and improvement of standards.** Essentially it is **a whole system/framework for improving quality through minimising risks by embracing patient safety through raising professional's awareness of their own accountability for excellence.** Clinical governance in our opinion is a system which should be able to demonstrate, in both primary, secondary, and acute care and services **that systems, process, practices, and procedures are in place guaranteeing clinical quality improvements at all levels of health and care provision.**

Given the backdrop of the above, **it is not surprising to see why worldwide clinical governance has become the mantra for all things related to safety, quality, governance, and improvement within the health and care sectors.** This may also **explain the popularity and integration of the term within many professional codes and standards for practice amongst the healthcare professions.** These include: Nursing [13], Medicine [14], Radiotherapy [15], Physiotherapy [16], Dentistry [17], Occupational Therapy [18] to name a few.

The key components, pillars, blocks, and/or concepts of clinical governance have advanced over-time. We believe this is in keeping with the primary aim of preserving person-centeredness, evidence-informed practice, safety, quality improvement, and learning and sharing from things that have gone well and/or not so well. It is also a sound indicator of data gathering, monitoring, improving, and changing practice when change is required. To engage with and apply the principle and concepts, it is important that you also understand the meaning of the term 'duty of candour'.

The need for the development of a statutory duty of candour, whereby a common health and care organisational culture and working environment is established for safeguarding and protecting health and care workers, patients/carers, and the public from harm and informing patient and families when things have gone wrong. For this to occur three core characteristics were identified. **'Openness':** having the ability to speak up freely without fear of reprisal and retaliation when highlighting concerns and/or alternatively sharing and celebrating success. **'Transparency':** communicating and sharing information about performance and outcomes in a truthfully honest way with healthcare workers, patients, and the public. **'Candour':** ensuring that, in the unfortunate situation where a patient is harmed by a healthcare worker and/or healthcare service, they or their legal next of kin are informed of the full facts. This should be at the earliest possible opportunity. An appropriate remedy should be afforded, wherein they are involved in any subsequent investigation/review that can facilitate learning and sharing. These stages of the process are essential in order to minimise recurrence of similar events; all this should occur regardless of a complaint and/or question raised regarding the situation. Where appropriate, a full apology should be offered, and detailed records maintained.

This is because safe health and care improvements and quality are dependent on the effectiveness of leaders and managers at all levels. All staff must be confident and competent with what sound governance principles mean and involve. This is because governance is and will remain a sound framework for safeguarding, protecting, and assuring the standards and quality of care in practice. Although we would argue that 'integrated governance' is an ideal term for highlighting the interconnectedness and interdependency of the various systems and processes akin to quality improvement, performance, and outcomes, many leaders and managers continue to embrace clinical governance because it is directly related to practice offering a useful framework for the provision of quality care, ongoing improvement, and outcomes. Furthermore, clinical governance is defined by McSherry and Pearce [19] as

> [...] a robust framework that acknowledges the importance of adopting a culture of shared accountability for sustaining and improving the quality of services and outcomes for both patients and staff.

Case Study 13.1: Applying the Principles and Components of Clinical Practice
Mrs D a 78-year-old lady was transferred from a nursing home to her local hospital for investigations and treatment into a sudden onset of swollen and painful joints. Mrs D on discharge back to her nursing home complained to her local hospital. The basis of her complaint was that following her admission on to the acute medical ward, a healthcare professional (could be a nurse, doctor, or any healthcare professional who undertakes adjustments to extend or expand their roles) was abrupt and insensitive when inserting a cannula into her right hand. This caused unnecessary pain, discomfort, and bruising because they tried several times to insert the cannula without success. Mrs D stated that it was not until a more experienced member of staff saw what was happening and took over this duty from the staff member that the cannula was inserted on the first attempt.

In recent years, health and care leaders/managers, on receiving this complaint, might have rushed into establishing how this had occurred and who was responsible for such an incident so that disciplinary procedures could be instigated. This reactionary approach to leadership/management does not bode well in the context of clinical governance that promotes an open and fair blame culture by the application of an authentic leadership/management style.

Let us explore how clinical governance may assist in overcoming this clinical incident associated with a health and care individuals' practice. Furthermore, let us support you in applying this to your own workplace and in enhancing your awareness of clinical governance.

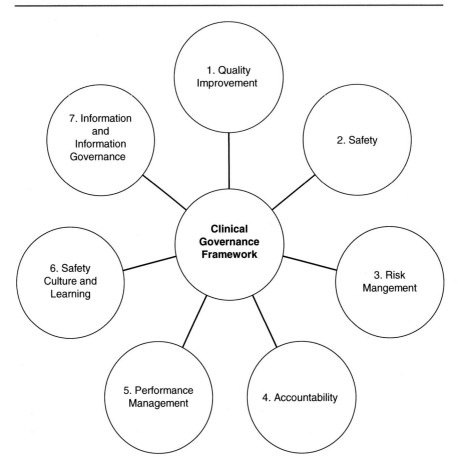

Fig. 13.2 Applying the key components of a clinical governance framework to health and care. *Note: Patient and carer partnerships should be established in order to elicit their experience through engagement and involvement throughout all the components. They should also be co-designers, producers, implementors, and evaluators of services*

Let us explore how you can apply the clinical governance framework to your health and care practice.

When looking at applying the clinical governance framework to the case study above, it is important to understand and learn about what the key components are and involve when investigating the incident. You will notice in Fig. 13.2 that the clinical governance framework comprises of a series of key components all having equal importance in the provision of safe, quality care and service. When applying this to Case Study 13.1, the following points emerge.

1. ***Quality Improvement:*** When looking at Mrs. D care, it is evident that this was not a quality experience on several fronts. A member of staff was rude, abrupt, and insensitive to her clinical needs and personal situation when inserting a

cannula. They failed to engage Mrs. D in the care processes and communicate with her during the procedure. In essence there was a failure to follow policy and guidance. To avoid this type of situation from occurring again, you and/or your organisation should familiarise yourself with the term 'clinical audit'. Clinical audit is a way that doctors, nurses, and other healthcare professionals can measure the quality of the care they offer. It allows them to compare their performance against a standard to see how they are doing and identify opportunities for improvement. Changes can then be made, followed by further audits to see if these changes have been successful.

2. *Safety:* Mrs. D safety was comprised by the member of staff failing to safeguard and protect the patient. A primary principle of any clinical governance framework is about ensuring the safety of our patients, colleagues, and the public. Essentially this should be our number one priority. Furthermore, it is about creating a safety culture/climate that is an important factor to achieve this goal. It is also about having a sound awareness of our working patterns, environment and openly speaking out if things do not and/or are not right (this is explored in more detail in the next section).

3. ***Risk management:*** In this situation risk management is about minimising risks to patients, health and care workers, and the public by identifying what works well and from what can and does go wrong during care and services, diagnostics, interventions, and treatment. In our opinion risk management is about creating a safety climate and culture where staff are constantly vigilant and are aware of how to recognise the concerns that influence the delivery of safe, quality care and services. This is essential in order to learn the lessons from any near misses, adverse or serious incidents/events and complaints. It is about investigating the situation and taking action to prevent recurrence and putting systems in place to reduce any further potential risks. Risk management is not just about looking for negative stories and experience but also about sharing accolades from, good experiences and outcomes when things have gone well.

4. ***Accountability:*** Generally defined, accountability is 'if you are accountable to someone for something that you do, you are responsible for it and must be prepared to justify your actions to that person'. Taking this definition into account and applying this to Mrs. D situation, accountability extends beyond the patient, to the employee, employer, the professions, and the law. When caring for Mrs. D, accountability primarily refers to four areas of your work. This is explained in Table 13.1.

   According to Table 13.1, health and care workers in exercising their duty of care are ultimately accountable *to the public*—through criminal law; *to the employer*—through contract law, contract of employment and job description and *to the patient*—through a duty of care, common and civil law.

5. **Performance Management:** In this situation, it is inextricably linked to accountability by ensuring you have the necessary knowledge, understanding, competence, and confidence to perform your role and responsibilities. In relation to Mrs. D situation, there was obviously a problem with the staff members performance. This could have been avoided. Firstly, by highlighting any areas of deficit

Table 13.1 Positioning accountability when caring for Mrs. D

Area	Theme	Rationale
1	*Employment*	As an individual as part of your role you have a duty of care and responsibility to safeguard and protect and provide quality work
2	*Ethics*	Ensuring you work collaboratively and effectively with other co-workers to deliver quality work, and to resolve potential work-related conflicts of interest, problems, ensuring fair and equitable treatment in the pursuit of safe compassionate quality care
3	*Professionally*	You are accountable for ensuring, enhancing, and maintaining high standards of practice within your health and care organisation. These standards ultimately impact on the performance, service provision and the achievement of key outcomes for oneself, others, the organisation, and profession(s). It is imperative you escalate any concerns that may compromise your ability to provide quality care
4	*Legally*	You are responsible for working within the law as well as within any health and safety, regulatory authorities, employment legislation, and professional regulations

Adapted from [20]

requiring attention immediately they arise, before and/or during your annual appraisal. This is essential in ensuring any supporting systems and frameworks can be developed for you. Secondly, it is about having regular supervision and access to statutory and mandatory training, i.e. fire, health and safety, infection prevention and data protection issues and systems in place for staff to speak openly and candidly about their place of work. Thirdly, it is about accessing ongoing education and training and continuous professional development in order to perform your role to its maximum potential. It is about safeguarding a duty of care where you have a moral or legal obligation to ensure the safety or wellbeing of yourself and others.

6. **Safety Culture and Learning:** At the heart of its many definitions is the fact that **'culture'** consists of the values, beliefs, and assumptions shared by occupational groups. These shared ways of thinking are then translated into common and repeated patterns of behaviour: patterns of behaviour that are in turn maintained and reinforced by rituals, ceremonies, and rewards of everyday organisational life [21]. What can we learn from reviewing the letters and themes akin to the word 'culture'? To demonstrate generality of the word culture, it is vital to explore the etymology of the word. Etymology in this instance refers to 'the origin and development of a word or affix' ([22], p. 296). In this situation it is associated with reviewing the meaning and symbols behind each letter! **C**—is akin to caring, care, compassion, commitment, courage, you care, i care, we care, they care, who cares, self-care and in creating a caring working environment. It is about designing and implementing systems and process to measure the impact and outcome of the care delivery systems. **U**—user focused centring on promoting patient [people]-centeredness through the utilisation of a facilitative approach to team working, collaboration, and partnership building. **L**—leadership will make a change happen. In this situation the task has only just

begun—"it is relatively easy to set out a vision, much harder to make it a reality" [12]. Authentic leadership openly acknowledges when improvement is required. **T**—teamwork, engagement through empowerment and the negotiation with everyone; partners, patients, professionals, etc… **U**—unlocking potential in order to facilitate staff and stakeholders along with patients to innovate and enterprise by embracing new ways of working, supporting professional practice and development and challenging self and others. **R**—responding and listening, actioning, and dealing with concerns, complaints, incidents, events and to facilitate the process of learning and sharing to avoid any reoccurrence of the situation. It is also about celebrating success and achievements and rewarding and recognising a job well done. **E**—evaluation is about embracing external scrutiny and review from regulators, professional bodies, and peer review.

7. *Information and Information Governance:* It is about ensuring data protection and confidentiality for patients, staff, and the public. Password protecting and ensuring staff have access to data that is commensurate with their role and responsibility. It is about recording and documenting information with factual accuracy.

According to Case Study 13.1 it is important to recognise that clinical governance is a framework designed to support health and care workers and organisations in providing safe, quality care and services. This is achieved by drawing together several key concepts all equally important in fostering an organisational culture and working environments that achieve the following:

- The systematic harmonisation of clinical and managerial/leadership roles and responsibilities associated with an individual's accountability and their practice.
- The improvement in a team dynamic, function and working by fostering more integrated team working in both the public and independent sectors.
- Striving for continuous quality improvement in all that health and care does by monitoring, changing, evaluating, and improving practice to safeguard and protect standards and people.
- The nurturing of a culture of continuous sharing and learning by placing a duty of care to improve individual, team, and organisational performance.
- Adopting a person-centeredness approach in all that we do is the heart of clinical governance [19].

13.5 Recognising, Responding, and Knowing How to Escalate Care Concerns for Both Patients and Staff

Raising a concern, escalating, and/or whistle blowing are terms often associated with a failure in either an individual and/or teams' performance [23]. Within a clinical governance framework, the emphasis is placed on safeguarding and protecting both the public and staff through fostering a culture and working environment in which safe quality care can flourish. This is founded on the principles of honesty, openness, transparency, and trust. Similarly, it is about sharing, learning, and celebrating when things go well and/or could be enhanced following an incident/event that may have emerged from whistleblowing.

If suboptimal care and/or services, a failure to safeguard and protect patients, staff and the public is evident it is imperative that we take action to highlight the concern. This could be done anonymously, by speaking out openly to your line manager and/or regulator. Speaking out is an undoubtedly a frightening and overwhelming situation for any individual to find themselves in. This is because it has the potential to impact upon their own general health and wellbeing along with those who will be under investigation and the service users/patients involved. Therefore, raising, and escalating issues/concerns requires confidence in knowing that you will be afforded the respect, dignity and if necessary, anonymity and confidentiality by your team and organisation. This is imperative in order to protect the individual, patient, and/or public. The important message for all health and care workers is the fact that you are doing nothing wrong by raising a concern. Speaking out is about safeguarding and protecting along with learning and sharing from a situation whether this is upheld or not. Excellence in practice requires the sharing and learning from incidents/events along with the celebration of achievement and success. Escalation is about 'safeguarding the health and wellbeing of those in your care' [24] along with safeguarding the health and wellbeing of staff and the public. We acknowledge there are numerous guidance, policies, and procedures explaining the systems and processes to raise concerns in your workplace. We would like to highlight the following.

(a) Raising concerns or issues should be encouraged and regarded as an integral part of safety, quality and governance systems and processes and therefore is an integral part of an individual's accountability.
(b) Escalation should be viewed as an immediate safeguarding quality mechanism.
(c) Escalation requires urgent actions and responses. This is essential in order to highlight areas where interventions, procedures, and interactions require improvement(s) along with individual attitudes, behaviours, and/or performance. It should not and cannot be left unchallenged.
(d) It is essential in order to avoid, improve, and minimise further risk and/or harm to the public and staff.
(e) When things go well at an individual, team, and/or organisational level, it is important for an organisation to openly acknowledge this regularly. This is because rewarding and celebrating success and achievements assists in creating an open and honest culture.
(f) A culture of openness, honesty, and trust requires a recognition of doing well. If an accolade is made about the experiences of a certain procedure or intervention these must also be openly encouraged and acknowledged.

We would like to draw your attention to a simple framework we developed that you may wish to consider in the future detailed in the suggested reading section.

13.6 Summary of Main Points

The contributing drivers that lead to and the continuing need for clinical governance in health and care can be attributed to issues with the following categories: political, professional, societal, economical.

Clinical governance is a framework for continual quality improvement of health and care services and staff by minimizing risks to safety and quality.

The future should focus on integrated health and care governance. This may be achieved by the harmonization of corporate governance and clinical governance across and between health and social care organizations and teams, and individuals.

We all have a duty and responsibility to escalate issues aligned to safeguarding and protecting patients, staff, and services.

13.7 Suggested Reading

Mannion, R.; Davies, H. (2018) Understanding organisational culture for healthcare quality improvement. BMJ Qual. Health Care, 363, 1136–1140.

McSherry, R., Pearce, P (2010) Clinical Governance a Guide to Implementation for Healthcare Professionals Wiley-Blackwell Publishers, Oxford.

McSherry R, McSherry W (2015) A model to support staff in raising concerns. Nursing Times; 111: 8, 15–17.

References

1. World Health Organization (2020) Aging and health. WHO, Geneva. https://www.who.int/news-room/fact-sheets/detail/ageing-and-health. Accessed 28 May 2020
2. Muir-Gray JA (1997) Evidence-based healthcare: how to make health policy and management decisions. Churchill Livingston: London.
3. Recio-Saucedo A, Dall'Ora C, Maruotti A et al (2018) What impact does nursing care left undone have on patient outcomes? Review of the literature. J Clin Nurs 27:2248–2259. http://eprints.bournemouth.ac.uk/30156/13/Recio-Saucedo_et_al-2018-Journal_of_Clinical_Nursing.pdf. Accessed 8 Oct 2019
4. Priestly C (2020) Second report on CQC following Whorlton Hall abuse scandal. The Northern Echo, 16 Dec 2020. Second report on CQC lfollowing Whorlton Hall abuse scandal | The Northern Echo. Accessed 4 Jan 2020
5. The Mid Staffordshire NHS Foundation Trust Public Inquiry (2013) Report of the Mid Staffordshire NHS Foundation Trust Public Inquiry, vol 3: Present and future annexes. The Stationery Office, London
6. France-Presse A (2017) South African scandal after nearly 100 mental health patients die. The Guardian. https://www.theguardian.com/world/2017/feb/01/south-african-scandal-after-nearly-100-mental-health-patients-die. Accessed 4 Jan 2021

7. Keegan G (2017) Cost of clinical negligence in trusts in parliament London. https://www.gilliankeegan.com/cost-clinical-negligence-trusts. Accessed 4 Jan 2021
8. National Health Service (2019) Population Health and the Population Health Management Programme NHS, London. Available on: https://www.england.nhs.uk/integratedcare/building-blocks/phm/. Accessed on 26 Mar 2021
9. National Health Service Improvement (2019) What we do. NHS, London. https://improvement.nhs.uk/about-us/what-we-do/. Accessed 4 Jan 2021
10. National Health Service Employers (2019) European working time directives. NHS, London. https://www.nhsemployers.org/~/media/Employers/Documents/SiteCollectionDocuments/WTD_FAQs_010609.pdf. Accessed 4 Jan 2021
11. Department of Health (1997) The new NHS modern and dependable, Department of Health. HMSO, London
12. Department of Health (2008) High Quality Care for All (Darzi Report). Department of Health, London
13. Royal College of Nursing (2020) Clinical governance. https://www.rcn.org.uk/clinical-topics/clinical-governance. Accessed 27 Sept 2020
14. General Medical Council (2020) Effective clinical governance for the medical profession. https://www.gmc-uk.org/registration-and-licensing/employers-medical-schools-and-colleges/effective-clinical-governance-for-the-medical-profession. Accessed 27 Sept 2020
15. The Society of Radiographers (2020) Clinical governance. https://www.sor.org/learning/document-library/independent-practitioners-standards-and-guidance/11-clinical-governance. Accessed 27 Sept 2020
16. West Hampstead Physiotherapy (2020) Clinical Governance Policy. http://physionw6.co.uk/clinical-governance-policy/. Accessed 27 Sept 2020
17. British Dental Association (2020) Safeguarding. https://www.bda.org/safeguarding. Accessed 1 Nov 2020
18. Royal College of Occupational Therapists (2015) Code of ethics and professional conduct. RCOT, London. file:///C:/Users/user/Downloads/Code%20of%20ethics%20update%202017.pdf. Accessed 1 Sept 2020
19. McSherry R, Pearce P (2010) Clinical governance a guide to implementation for healthcare professionals. Wiley-Blackwell Publishers, Oxford
20. National Health Service Education for Scotland (2016) Professionalism and Professional Accountability in Clinical Skills Practice: Available on: http://www.csmen.scot.nhs.uk/media/1318/professionalism_and_professional_accountability.pdf. Accessed 26 Mar 2021
21. Mannion R, Davies H (2018) Understanding organisational culture for healthcare quality improvement. BMJ Qual Health Care 363:1136–1140
22. Collins W (1987) Collins Universal English Dictionary. Readers Union Ltd, Glasgow
23. Department of Health (2010) How to implement and review whistleblowing arrangements in your organisation Social Partnership Forum & Public Concern at Work, London
24. Nursing and Midwifery Council (2013) Raising concerns: guidance for nurses and midwives. NMC, London

Contemporary Developments

14

Mari S. Berge

Contents

14.1 Learning Objectives

- Explore how to plan care to support the person's resources
- Understand how various telecare solutions require different cognitive interactions
- Appreciate why older people should be involved in designing their own care solutions

M. S. Berge (✉)
Faculty of Health and Social Sciences, Western Norway University of Applied Sciences, Bergen, Norway
e-mail: mber@hvl.no, Mari.Synnove.Berge@hvl.no

© Springer Nature Switzerland AG 2021
W. McSherry et al. (eds.), *Understanding Ageing for Nurses and Therapists*,
Perspectives in Nursing Management and Care for Older Adults,
https://doi.org/10.1007/978-3-030-40075-0_14

14.2   Introduction

When focusing on the contemporary developments in today's services for older people it is necessary to pay attention to the resources possessed by today's older generation. People live longer and are healthier and more socially active than previously [1]. However, a general feature is often to present older people as being solely dependent passive receivers of care. The biological changes due to age differ widely and decrease in physical and mental capacity are only loosely associated with a person's age in years [2]. Many older people have unused resources and given the right opportunities they may make better use of these to increase their quality of life [3]. Remaining and living safely in one's own home is not only the policy in several governments, it is the goal of older people in general as it may support them with healthy ageing [4, 5]. To understand the best way to enable older people to remain at home their voice must receive attention, as it is the fundamental aspect of all health and social care: the persons in question are the experts of their own lives.

The demographic prospects forecast a rise in the gap between health service providers and those in need for their services and thus this entails a transfer of more responsibilities to the relatives. Relatives often provide different kinds of assistance to older persons, however, regarding relatives as "carers" might conceal kinship and cause confusion of roles [1]. In this chapter, the term *relative* is thus preferred instead of *carer* even if the relative has an additional role as carer for the older person. Relatives account for many hours of (often unpaid) assistance and their contribution is essential for sustaining the care services.

Healthcare services are transforming from being institutional care to becoming more based on home care, and technology offers possibilities at home that are otherwise difficult to achieve [3, 6]. Several research projects emphasise how correctly adjusted telecare improve older people's abilities to remain safe in their own home for longer [3, 7, 8]. Different terms appear in research regarding the use of technology in care settings and the ambiguity in terms complicates comparisons and reviewing [8, 9]. By using technology an older person may first and foremost rely on their own physical and cognitive resources instead of relying on assistance [10]. However, implementing technology in care might challenge how health and social care professionals work. I will address these topics by using examples and findings from a recent telecare project conducted in Norway [9].

Reflective Question
What is your understanding of telecare and assistive technologies? If at all—how do you differentiate between these terms?

14.3 Telecare: A Necessary Competence Within Contemporary Care

People live longer and despite many experiencing significant deterioration in health, a large number have little change in their physical and mental capacities [2]. Treating people as a homogeneous group tends to mask differences [11] while the varieties in older people's functioning are increasing and thus the diversity in their perceived needs is expected to expand [2].

Technology to enable older people to manage everyday life autonomously is receiving increased attention from researchers and policymakers [6]. In this chapter I use telecare as defined by the Department of Health (United Kingdom) [12]:

> Personal and environmental sensors in the home that enable people to remain safe and independent in their own home for longer. 24 hour monitoring ensures that, should an event occur, the information is acted upon immediately and the most appropriate response put in train.

This perspective on technology, named telecare, emphasises how the person *is not required to interact*, and thus offers different possibilities and challenges from technologies that entail interaction. One well-known device that requires interaction is the social alarm, which has a button that the users must push to alert when they need assistance. To activate the social alarm you must (1) understand the concept of pushing the button for it to alert, (2) you must consider yourself being in a situation to which you need assistance, and (3) you must have the social alarm within reach when you need it. Nurses report how older people frequently do not use the social alarm due to missing one or more of these requirements [9].

Contrary to social alarms that require the persons themselves to assess a situation when it occurs, telecare requires that the conditions have been assessed in forehand. Each situation needs thorough assessment by a nurse or therapist in close cooperation with the persons that are to receive telecare in their home, and their relatives. Telecare consists typically of various sensors that are wireless connected to a home unit. One sensor might have different functions from another similar sensor as they might require different response. In one situation, a movement or pressure sensor may cause the lights to turn on, in another to turn them off.

Older people appear to be reluctant to display their lack of cooping as they want to refrain from burdening others [13]. In general, they want to remain living in their own home [4, 5, 9, 14]; however, they prioritise safety to independence [15]. Many fear becoming a burden to others (relatives) if they do not comply with well-meant suggestions of moving to an institution when their safety is at risk.

To demonstrate the importance of remaining at home, I will use examples from a resent telecare project where service users, relatives and service providers give voice to what is important for them in their everyday lives. The following cases and solutions are constructed from several actual experiences from my research [9]:

Case 1: Living an Independent Life at Risk

Olivia is 88 years old and loves to be independent and mobile. She is a widow of 20 years and is proud to manage on her own. Olivia goes by bus to the nearby village where she does her shopping, sees her GP and joins in several activities and enjoys the company of her friends. She has a variety of medical conditions among these are diabetes, a minor heart condition and dizziness. Her main concern is the dizziness that occurs when she changes position from lying to standing, especially at night when she has to visit the bathroom. Olivia has no problems with managing her medication. She lives in her own house where she has lived since they were married 65 years ago. The ground floor contains the entrance, the kitchen and the living room, while her bedroom and the bathroom are on the second floor. She therefore must use the stairs several times a day. *"The stairs keep me fit as a fiddle"*, she says. According to Olivia the stairs seldom cause any trouble; however, due to a couple of incidents where she fell and injured herself, her daughter Sandra holds a different opinion. *"She fell on the stairs last winter when she came back from the village. Fortunately, I came shortly after but that was sheer coincidence. What might have happened if I hadn't come? She was not able to get up or to move"*.

Olivia receives no help from community care and she reject any offer of help. *"I have always managed by myself and I enjoy being able to rise, eat and shower according to my own schedule and not following that of others"*. Olivia and Sandra speak on the phone every night before bedtime but Sandra is worried, as she is aware of her mother's dizziness and knows that she needs to negotiate the steep stairs to go to bed and also to use the bathroom a couple of times during the night. Sandra respects and understands Olivia's decision to remain living in her home but still discusses the advantages of moving to a care centre. The situation now threatens their relationship; Olivia feels that her way of life has become a burden to her daughter, which she in turn feels increasingly burdening and as a result is diminishing her joy of living independently.

The above situation illustrates how many older people experience that their wish to continue living autonomously in their own home, may challenge their relatives' peace of mind. Thus, the older person might refrain from being open about difficulties as they seek to avoid provoking further discussions about moving. Several of my interviewees emphasised how they valued being autonomous and planning their days and life according to their own preferences [9].

The relatives in my interviews usually had caring obligations in various ways; however, they regarded themselves as daughters and sons and not as carers, as did their parents. For further reading: Judith Phillips [1] comprehensively discusses the mix up of roles between relatives being carers.

In the above case, Olivia risks losing her home and her life as she knows it if she wants to remain in a good relationship with her daughter. Sandra hates herself for imposing her worries on her mother and dislikes having to encourage her to move. Mother and daughter realise that their ongoing discussion is far from fruitful and potentially leading to a deterioration in their relationship. They therefore agree to discuss the issue with the home care nurse, and they make an appointment for her to meet them in Olivia's house.

14.4   The Nursing Process in Telecare Assessment

When the community care nurse arrives, she listens attentively to both women aiming to understand and assess the situation from their diverse perspectives. Firstly, she emphasises how the activities in Olivia's everyday life improve her abilities to remain home and meticulously highlights her resources. Then she encourages Olivia to present her challenges. She includes both women in analysing the situation, they agree upon there being an issue with safety but that abandoning her home is too high a cost for Olivia. The nurse informs about telecare that is part of the new service offered by the community care team. She explains briefly the main functioning of the different sensors and gives them a pamphlet for further reading. Olivia is reluctant to be included as a service user despite wanting the safety that telecare offers. The nurse explains how the various sensors might go directly via the response centre to her relatives, for example to her daughter Sandra, without involving the community care. She does however advocate the benefits of including home care for safety reasons if the relatives are unable to respond. Likewise, she informs how Olivia may benefit from being included in the local government emergency plans in case of severe situations. She illustrates this by explaining how the local government maintains safety in situations caused by severe weather conditions that occur frequently during the winter season.

Together they discuss the situation and agree on Olivia's need being to maintain safety at home due to her risk of falling. The nurse suggests the following solutions: bed and chair sensors connected to light sensors, two movement sensors and smoke detector in both floors.

The bed sensor detects the presence or absence of pressure. Olivia usually needs 10–15 min when she visits the bathroom at night. They agree on the sensor alerting if she is away more than 30 min, as she occasionally needs some more time. They discuss which time the sensor should activate and agree on 11 pm, as Olivia usually prefers to go to bed between 10 and 11 pm. The bed sensor connects to a light that activates with absence of pressure. Thus, when Olivia leaves the bed, a light will turn on and help her to find her way and avoid stumbling. Should Olivia be absent from bed for more than 30 min the response centre is alerted and may contact her to further investigate the situation. This check includes negotiating with Olivia whether she needs assistance from Sandra who wishes to be summoned as she lives quite close. Olivia usually rises at 8 am in the morning but some nights she has trouble sleeping and goes downstairs to sit comfortably in her favourite chair. The nurse assessed how the nights usually were; however, she paid particular attention to any irregularities, as these often cause false alerts. Therefore, she recommended an additional pressure sensor in Olivia's favourite chair. This sensor also connects to a light but in this situation, it turns the light on when pressure occurs as Olivia likes to knit when she cannot sleep and thus needs the light. They also agree on one movement sensor in the living room and one in the kitchen. These will alert when movement is not detected in any of the two rooms for 4 h during daytime. To enable this solution Olivia will have to inform the system if she leaves the house as well as when she returns. She therefore must deactivate the system when she leaves and activate it when she returns. Since Olivia has no cognitive problems, she expects no problems in including this into her habitual routines when leaving the house. Finally, the nurse suggests changing the smoke detectors to new ones integrated in the system that will alert directly to the fire department.

In addition, the nurse suggests that Olivia receives a social alarm that she can wear around her wrist or as a pendant around her neck and activate if a situation occurs or if she feels unsafe. Politely Olivia declined this offer, as she thinks herself sufficiently safeguarded with the less conspicuous sensors that are hidden under her mattress and under the chair cushion or appear like an ordinary intruder alarm. The smoke detectors are almost like her old ones. Sandra tried to argue for increased safety, but Olivia did not want to display that she needed extra support. She had seen the sensors as the nurse brought them when visiting, and Olivia was content that these sensors would not make her "feel old and frail" as this deviated from her self-image. The social alarm however did not comply with her self-image.

Olivia and her daughter received information and explanation when the nurse and the technician implemented the telecare service. Later there had to be some adjustments as Olivia often went to bed later than 11 pm. Both women were satisfied with the "false alarms" as they experienced it to demonstrate that the system was reliable. One year later, they were happy and Sandra had peace of mind as she said, *"If Mum needs assistance I <u>know</u> the system will alert because we had a few unintended alarms, which actually had a quite calming effect as I felt telecare proved to be reliable"*.

Case 2: In Risk of Moving from the Known to the Unknown
Lisa is 90 years, a widow of more than 40 years, she has dementia and lives alone in her small semi-detached apartment. She has a small sheltered garden, which she accesses from her living room. She was in a nursing home for 6 weeks after a hip fracture and both she and her family (two sons and a daughter) were unhappy with that solution. Lisa has a heartfelt desire to remain in her little home where she enjoys gardening and pottering about seeing to everything and nothing. Lisa has problems with taking care of herself, and her family understands that she cannot be left all alone. She refuses to let anybody clean her house and do her laundry. However, she allows a few nurses to assist her when showering, nevertheless reluctantly.

Lisa accepts to attend the day care centre as she meets some old childhood friends there. She has dinner when she is there and appears to join in with her friends. Recently, the neighbours have expressed their worry as they have observed Lisa outdoors in her slippers late in the evening. The family feel they are in a desperate situation, as they have to choose between two hopeless situations, forcing Lisa to move or leave her at home exposed to hazards. Relying on the neighbours observations, the family fears that Lisa leaves her home during night and gets lost and/or harms herself. Both situations, forcing Lisa to move or leave her on her own at home, will cause misery to all involved.

The relatives discuss the situation with the nurse without including their mother. Together with the nurse, they conclude that the main objective is that Lisa is happy without being exposed to hazards. Documentation from the previous stay in the nursing home and the relatives' descriptions of the changes in Lisa's mood and behaviour give the nurse data to help in her assessment of the situation. She explains the change in policy to help people remain in their home and emphasise that they might try to include telecare in the services for a while before admitting Lisa to nursing home.

Together the nurse and the relatives agree that Lisa will receive home care to help her wash and get dressed every morning. They will make an effort to keep the number of different nurses visiting her to a minimum and try to use the few nurses Lisa accepts when helping her showering. They will increase her number of days at the day care centre from two to three and provide breakfast and dinner while she is there. The family will do her shopping and laundry and the cleaner will come once a week when Lisa attends the day care centre. In addition, the relatives want to have door sensors installed. These will alert if Lisa leaves home during evening or night. If Lisa opens the main door just to peek out while remaining indoors, she will not set off any alarm as a movement sensor overrules the door sensor. However, if she leaves the premises the home care services will be notified. They agreed on a "silent alarm", which means that there will not be any sound to scare Lisa. The alarm summons the home care team. An important consideration when using a silent alarm is how to explain your arrival as a response to the alarm as the person (with dementia) will not be aware of any alarm, and might worry. The home care team are there to assist him/her, which is a plausible reason to give. Lisa's relatives would also use a movement sensor that would alert if there were movement during night to document whether Lisa was restless during night. They agreed not to visit her during night but use that documentation to inform the nurse to make her more aware when visiting in the morning. The nurse explained the option to install a camera that could detect whether Lisa was in bed, had fallen, etc. by using blurred images combined with an alert. They discussed this possibility, but the relatives felt it being too obtrusive and wanted to try without.

Lisa remained home for almost a year with this solution. Telecare was adjusted according to minor changes and after a few months, the relatives agreed to include the camera to check on Lisa if the movement sensors showed activity during the night. The joint solution from community care and relatives gave Lisa the necessary help and telecare increased her safety, as she would receive assistance if necessary. The door sensor documented that Lisa never went out in the evening but remained home. She enjoyed her life at home but due to pneumonia, she was hospitalised and died. Her relatives were content with her being able to remain as autonomously for her last year.

14.5 What These Two Cases Demonstrate

These two cases show in different ways how contemporary nursing will need to cooperate with the persons themselves and their relatives in tailoring better individual support including community care and telecare. The nurse/therapist must carry out and manage the assessment according to the nursing process. The nurse/therapist will need to have a thorough understanding of how telecare works, what it does and what it does not do, as they will need to guide the implementation to individual resources and needs. As an example, Olivia receives a pressure sensor in her bed while Lisa does not. This sensor does not discriminate which pressure activates it, just that a pressure occurs. The nurse refrain from using the pressure sensor with Lisa, because she knows that people with dementia might choose a different place to sleep or have various changes in their sleep pattern. The contemporary nurse needs knowledge of technology in addition to their nursing skills and they must be able to help users and their relatives in finding the better solution to match their needs.

Ethical issues might arise when using telecare, and ethical considerations must be part of any assessment and every situation. General ethical issues that often arise as they also do in the above cases are:

- Who benefit from the telecare solution?
- May telecare cause less contact with community care and may that increase loneliness?
- Is it justifiable that older people remain living at home when they cannot take properly care of themselves?

We should remember that using new solutions often challenge our ethical conscience more than those that are part of our routines without necessarily being less ethical. We need to make ethical considerations with any solution with and without including telecare as part of the service.

> **Reflective Exercise**
> - Discuss the above cases from an ethical perspective.
> - Think of a situation from your own practice and consider various solutions with and without telecare. Who do you need to involve in the assessments and which goals and needs will you emphasise and prioritise? Which information will you need for being able to find a better solution and how will you know which solution to choose?
> - What reasons did you identify for including and not including telecare in your care?

14.6 The Voice of Older People in Research

Providing contemporary care will include using current technology, like telecare, however each situation needs individual assessment. Different people have different needs, demands and expectations towards using telecare. Whether these are conflicting or consistent is likely to affect the over-all results. Bowes and McColgan [6] highlight that research and evaluations have in fact privileged the service providers' point of view and thus reducing the persons using the service merely to a recipient of the service. We know from several research projects that if the technology does not match the users' needs, they may stop using the solution [9, 16]. In an ageing population, it is crucial to gain insight by listening to older people in designing solutions aiming to match their actual needs in health and social care, no matter the character of the services. This topic receives increased attention and when the researchers prepare for the older people to participate, they are both able and willing to give valuable input [17]. When developing telecare solutions it is essential to listen to experiences from older people as there are differences between what people *think* about a solution they have not tried and what they actually *experience* from using it [3, 16]. When people experience benefits from telecare, their opinion regarding advantages and disavantages also appear to be more nuanced [18]. However, people in general, independent of age are reluctant to use any device if it marks them as helpless in any way [19]. Therefore, people should be given the opportunity to try telecare, to experience it as part of their life before deciding upon a solution [9].

Another important issue to consider is who the designers are that design artefacts and solutions for older people. Many designers are younger people with little experience or understanding from older people's perspectives. Research has documented how design intended for older people actually excluded the targeted users (older people) due to the design being unsuitable for them [10]. Experiences from involving people with dementia in developing devices determined for their use provided useful information during the development process [20]. Including older people in research is both necessary and important when designing contemporary health and social care services to their benefit [3, 6, 17, 20].

14.7   Caring for the Carer

As explained in the beginning of this chapter, I use the term "relatives" even if they take on the role as "carer" [1]. Relatives are essential in supporting older people to remain living in their own home [21]. Relatives very often take on a role of caring and taking responsibility for a variety of tasks [22]. They usually attend to needs without perceiving their role to be changed from that of being a daughter, a spouse and a grandchild [1]. Carlsen and Lundberg [22] found that relatives perceived their effort as carer both as a duty and as a choice and thus a meaningful task. Nevertheless, when people are in a situation where they hold responsibility for another person, they experience this becoming a burden over time [21]. Relatives are known to contribute to several hours of assistance but often experience the "not knowing" to be among the most stressful [9, 21]. Caring for the relatives that are in a position of being a carer needs explicit focus when planning the care solution.

When health and social care policies are aiming for more people to remain living in their own home, and the demographics show a continuing ageing populations, it is natural to conclude that the input from relatives will need to increase and will remain an important resource in the provision of future health and social care. Health and social care personnel are usually attentive to the possible strain relatives have when taking on caring responsibilities. However, relatives might play an increasing role in the joint planning for older people to remain living at home. It is important to take good care of these essential resources. Research indicates that traditional arrangements in respite for carers are beneficial [21]. In addition, research emphasises that it is important for the relatives that their effort is acknowledged and appreciated by health and social care personnel [22].

Research from newer care solutions, like telecare, demonstrates that when relatives trust the telecare solution, they express that they have a greater peace of mind [3]. However, for the relatives and the service users to trust telecare, the nurses must have made a thorough assessment of the situation and configured the solution according to the actual needs and resources [8, 9].

14.8   Summary

This chapter reinforces how the field of nursing and social care are changing in line with the demographic of an ageing population. People are living longer and have resources that need to be both recognised and utilised in future care planning. Telecare provides a new dimension in care that when used correctly may support remaining resources in beneficial ways for the older person and their relatives. Positive experiences from using telecare depend to a high degree on how well the nurse or allied health professional assesses the situation and thereafter manages to engage with the user and their relatives to design and apply a tailored care solution. In contemporary and future care, the relatives are essential resources that need to be respected and acknowledged. To provide optimal care solutions that utilise and support resources the involved persons need to be involved and thus they are able to share their experiences and knowledge of ageing.

14.9 Suggested Reading

Berge MS. Telecare - where, when, why and for whom does it work? A realist evaluation of a Norwegian project. Journal of Rehabilitation and Assistive Technologies Engineering. 2017;4:1–10.

Holroyd-Leduc J, Resin J, Ashley L, Barwich D, Elliott J, Huras P, et al. Giving voice to older adults living with frailty and their family caregivers: engagement of older adults living with frailty in research, health care decision making, and in health policy. Research Involvement and Engagement. 2016;2 (1):23.

Peek STM, Wouters EJM, van Hoof J, Luijkx KG, Boeije HR, Vrijhoef HJM. Factors influencing acceptance of technology for aging in place: A systematic review? International Journal of Medical Informatics. 2014 Apr;83 (4):235–48.

References

1. Phillips J (2007) Care. Polity Press, Cambridge
2. WHO (2015) World report on ageing and health: World Health Organization
3. Berge MS (2017) Telecare - where, when, why and for whom does it work? A realist evaluation of a Norwegian project. J Rehabilit Assist Technol Eng 4:1–10
4. Bergland A, Slettebø Å (2014) Health capital in everyday life of the oldest old living in their own homes. Ageing Soc 1:1–20
5. Sixsmith J, Sixsmith A, Fänge AM, Naumann D, Kucsera C, Tomsone S et al (2014) Healthy ageing and home: the perspectives of very old people in five European countries. Soc Sci Med 106:1–9
6. Bowes AM, McColgan GM (2013) Telecare for older people: promoting Independence, participation, and identity. Res Aging 35(1):32–49
7. Berge MS (2016) Telecare acceptance as sticky entrapment: a realist review. Gerontechnology 15(2):98–108
8. Karlsen C, Ludvigsen MS, Moe CE, Haraldstad K, Thygesen E (2017) Experiences of community-dwelling older adults with the use of telecare in home care services: a qualitative systematic review. JBI Database System Rev Implement Rep 15(12):2913–2980
9. Berge MS (2017) Challenges and possibilities in telecare: realist evaluation of a Norwegian telecare project 2017
10. Cartwright C, Wade R, Shaw K (2011) The impact of Telehealth and Telecare on clients of the Transition Care Program (TCP): Southern Cross University-Aged Services Learning & Research Collaboration
11. Farquhar M (1995) Elderly people's definitions of quality of life. Soc Sci Med 41(10):1439–1446
12. Department of Health (UK) (2011) Whole system demonstrator programme: headline findings – December 2011. Department of Health, London
13. Kofod J (2008) Becoming a nursing home resident. Unpublished doctoral dissertation, Technical University of Denmark, Copenhagen
14. Haak M, Fänge A, Iwarsson S, Dahlin IS (2007) Home as a signification of independence and autonomy: experiences among very old Swedish people. Scand J Occup Ther 14(1):16–24

15. Fonad E, Wahlin T-BR, Heikkila K, Emami A (2006) Moving to and living in a retirement home: focusing on elderly people's sense of safety and security. J Hous Elder 20(3):45–60
16. Peek STM, Wouters EJM, van Hoof J, Luijkx KG, Boeije HR, Vrijhoef HJM (2014 Apr) Factors influencing acceptance of technology for aging in place: a systematic review? Int J Med Inform 83(4):235–248
17. Holroyd-Leduc J, Resin J, Ashley L, Barwich D, Elliott J, Huras P et al (2016) Giving voice to older adults living with frailty and their family caregivers: engagement of older adults living with frailty in research, health care decision making, and in health policy. Res Involve Engage 2(1):23
18. Boise L, Wild K, Mattek N, Ruhl M, Dodge HH, Kaye J (2013) Willingness of older adults tvo share data and privacy concerns after exposure to unobtrusive in-home monitoring. Gerontechnology 11(3):428
19. Erber JT, Szuchman LT (2015) Great myths of aging. Wiley, Chichester
20. McCabe L, Innes A (2013) Supporting safe walking for people with dementia: user participation in the development of new technology. Geron 12(1):4–15
21. Greenwood N, Habibi R, Mackenzie A (2012) Respite: carers' experiences and perceptions of respite at home. BMC Geriatr 12(1):42
22. Carlsen B, Lundberg K (2018) 'If it weren't for me…': perspectives of family carers of older people receiving professional care. Scand J Caring Sci 32(1):213–221

Afterword

There has been a raft of new books of late on social aspects of ageing related to health professions particularly in relation to nursing and therapy. These have fallen into two main expositions: theory and practice; a demarcation of the 'thinkers' and the 'doers' of social research in relation to nursing and therapy. It would be fair to say that there is a contradiction which lies at the heart of contemporary health professions. On the one hand, there is research which is data rich but theory poor. Equally, on the other hand, there is research which is theory rich but data poor. Overcoming this is a difficult task. The answer is here. This is the first book I have read in a very long time to overcome this duality by presenting an impressive theoretically grounded understanding of rich empirical data for theory, policy and practice.

Before this book came along, for many years, a form of academic and institutional ageism prevented the cultivation and dissemination of research on older people. This was because of the intense interest on life-course studies focusing on youth by practitioners, public policy makers and academic researchers. (Although of course this is not to deny the importance or significance of that group of people at one end of the life-course.)

Related to this, both historically and contemporaneously, any suggestion of 'age' has instantly been ascribed to children, which then adds to the marginalisation and invisibility of older people as a 'hidden' age group within academic research and further reifies the holistic understanding of 'age' as a social characteristic.

It has taken many years for public policy makers finally to turn their attention to the 'ageing population' (comprised, ironically, of an increasingly visible group of older people, despite there having been hidden in the academic research).

This is an outstanding text that gives the ability to shed light on the importance of valuing older people and is indispensable in this regard. This book should provide sensitivity to policy makers and carers in recognising that older people are people with human rights and dignity. Until recently there has been a lack of basic training programmes or undergraduate and postgraduate courses in working with older people that had a text that has much depth and breadth that is covered by the material

© Springer Nature Switzerland AG 2021
W. McSherry et al. (eds.), *Understanding Ageing for Nurses and Therapists*,
Perspectives in Nursing Management and Care for Older Adults,
https://doi.org/10.1007/978-3-030-40075-0

by McSherry et al. Because of the overwhelming focus on working with children, there have been periodic episodes of inhumanity against older people which is known today as 'elder abuse'. This is not just a Western phenomenon but a global issue that affects all nations, including the UK. It had been forgotten that older people actually are people.

Due to the above, there was also a chronic shortage of research and knowledge for academics, carers, families and health care professionals on the vulnerabilities of older people, whether living at home or in a care home. This outstanding book comes at an ideal time when thinking on ageing requires an urgent reconstruction. This book provides a challenging context to understanding ageing, and the broad and historical range of the book is utterly compelling. The book is theoretically and methodologically robust and is a 'must-read' for qualitative researchers interested in understanding and applying conceptual and theoretical models of ageing to social practice with older people.

The ability to shed light on the importance of valuing older people is indispensable in this regard. This book should provide sensitivity to policy makers and carers in recognising that older people are people with human rights and dignity. Unfortunately, recent research on the very notion of 'ageing populations' has lumped 'older people' into a single undifferentiated category, as though population constructs based on old age are not differentiated by 'race', gender, sexuality, disability, class or history.

Engaging in research with older people is important to make researchers and practitioners understand the unique biographies, and this book makes a strong case for that. There is also a need to move beyond the current academic literature on caring for older people in care settings and persuade policy makers, researchers and carers to think deep and act on what it means to be cared about and cared for as an older person.

This book gives a united message on the importance of actually listening to and engaging with older people as service providers in order to address social divisions head on, so that public policy makers, carers and academic researchers can all learn from older people and their experiences: the real experts.

The book is also a tour de force in terms of development of social theory. I would suggest that this book will be extensively cited and deserves to be at the forefront of the sociology of caring literature for decades to come.

Jason L. Powell
Chester University
Chester, UK

Printed in the United States
by Baker & Taylor Publisher Services